Gastric Cancer

Contemporary Issues in Cancer Imaging

A Multidisciplinary Approach

Series Editor

Rodney H. Reznek
Cancer Imaging, St Bartholomew's Hospital, London

Editorial Adviser

Janet E. Husband
Diagnostic Radiology, Royal Marsden Hospital, Surrey

Current titles in the series

Cancer of the Ovary
Lung Cancer
Colorectal Cancer
Carcinoma of the Kidney
Carcinoma of the Esophagus
Carcinoma of the Bladder
Squamous Cell Cancer of the Neck
Prostate Cancer
Interventional Radiological Treatment of Liver Tumors
Pancreatic Cancer

Forthcoming titles in the series

Primary Carcinomas of the Liver
Breast Cancer

Gastric Cancer

Edited by

Richard M. Gore

Series Editor

Rodney H. Reznek

Editorial Adviser

Janet E. Husband

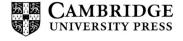

CAMBRIDGE
UNIVERSITY PRESS

CAMBRIDGE UNIVERSITY PRESS
Cambridge, New York, Melbourne, Madrid, Cape Town, Singapore,
São Paulo, Delhi, Dubai, Tokyo

Cambridge University Press
The Edinburgh Building, Cambridge CB2 8RU, UK

Published in the United States of America by Cambridge University Press, New York

www.cambridge.org
Information on this title: www.cambridge.org/9780521513838

© Cambridge University Press 2010

First published 2010

Printed in the United Kingdom at the University Press, Cambridge

A catalogue record for this publication is available from the British Library

Library of Congress Cataloguing in Publication data
Gastric cancer / [edited by] Richard M. Gore.
    p. ; cm. – (Contemporary issues in cancer imaging)
Includes bibliographical references and index.
ISBN 978-0-521-51383-8 (Hardcopy)   1. Stomach–Cancer.   I. Gore, Richard M.
II. Title   III. Series: Contemporary issues in cancer imaging.
[DNLM: 1. Stomach Neoplasms. WI 320 G2549 2010]
RC280.S8G3755 2010
616.99'433–dc22   2009035031

ISBN 978-0-521-51383-8 Hardback

Contents

Contributors

Marshall S. Baker
Department of Surgery
Division of Surgical Oncology
NorthShore University Health System
University of Chicago
Evanston, IL
USA

Malcolm M. Bilimoria
Department of Surgery
Evanston Northwestern Healthcare
University of Chicago
Evanston, IL
USA

Cheri L. Canon
Department of Radiology
University of Alabama Medical Center
Birmingham, AL
USA

Chiao-Yun Chen
Department of Radiology
Kaohsiung Medical University
Department of Medical Imaging
Kaohsiung, Taiwan

Richard M. Gore
Department of Radiology
NorthShore University Health System
University of Chicago
Evanston, IL
USA

Curtis R. Hall
Department of Pathology
NorthShore University Health System
University of Chicago
Evanston, IL
USA

Janardan D. Khandekar
Department of Medicine
Evanston Northwestern Healthcare
University of Chicago
Evanston, IL
USA

Melin Khandekar
Harvard Radiation Oncology Program,
Harvard Medical School,
Boston, MA
USA

Jung Hoon Kim
Body Imaging Section
Department of Radiology
University of Iowa Hospital and Clinics
Iowa City, IA
USA

Marc S. Levine
Department of Radiology
Hospital of the University of Pennsylvania
Philadelphia, PA
USA

Mark E. Lockhart
Department of Radiology
University of Alabama Medical Center
Birmingham, AL
USA

Hiroyuki Osawa
Department of Internal Medicine
Division of Gastroenterology
and
Jichi Medical University
Shimotsuke, Tochigi
Japan

Mark S. Talamonti
Department of Surgery
Division of Surgical Oncology
NorthShore University Health System

University of Chicago
Evanston, IL
USA

Hironori Yamamoto
Department of Internal Medicine
Division of Gastroenterology
Jichi Medical University
Shimotsuke, Tochigi
Japan

Kenjiro Yasuda
Department of Gastroenterology
Kyoto Second [Red] Cross Hospital
Haruobi-cho, Kamigyo-ku
Kyoto
Japan

Huan Zhang
Department of Radiology
Ruijin Hospital
Shanghai
China

Series Foreword

Imaging has become pivotal in all aspects of the management of patients with cancer. At the same time it is acknowledged that optimal patient care is best achieved by a multidisciplinary team approach. The explosion of technological developments in imaging over the past years has meant that all members of the multidisciplinary team should understand the potential applications, limitations and advantages of all the evolving and exciting imaging techniques. Equally, to understand the significance of the imaging findings and to contribute actively to management decisions and to the development of new clinical applications for imaging, it is critical that the radiologist should have sufficient background knowledge of different tumors. Thus the radiologist should understand the pathology, the clinical background, the therapeutic options, and prognostic indicators of malignancy.

Contemporary Issues in Cancer Imaging – A Multidisciplinary Approach aims to meet the growing requirement for radiologists to have detailed knowledge of the individual tumors in which they are involved in making management decisions. A series of single subject issues, each of which will be dedicated to a single tumor site and edited by recognized expert guest editors, will include contributions from basic scientists, pathologists, surgeons, oncologists, radiologists, and others.

While the series is written predominantly for the radiologist, it is hoped that individual issues will contain sufficient varied information so as to be of interest to all medical disciplines and to other health professionals managing patients with cancer. As with imaging, advances have occurred in all these disciplines related to cancer management and it is our fervent hope that this series, bringing together expertise from such a range of related specialties, will not only promote the understanding and rational application of modern imaging but will also help to achieve the ultimate goal of improving outcomes of patients with cancer.

Rodney H. Reznek

Preface to Gastric Cancer

Gastric adenocarcinoma is the second most common cancer in the world. Nearly one million new cases of this tumor develop annually and well over 700 000 individuals die from this neoplasm each year. In Asia, gastric cancer accounts for 31% of all cancer incidence cases in men and for 22% in women. Because of aggressive screening programs, gastric cancer is often found at an earlier, potentially curable stage in Asia. In the West, this tumor is usually diagnosed in its later stages and the prognosis is grim. Indeed, even with modern diagnostic and treatment methods, only 10% of patients in the West are alive within five years of diagnosis.

Improvements in overall survival of patients with gastric cancer can only be achieved by earlier diagnosis and by tailored therapeutic strategies that are based on histologic tumor type, tumor location, tumor stage at the time of presentation, and the physiologic status of the patient. The purpose of this book is to provide a state of the art, integrated diagnostic and therapeutic approach to patients with this lethal neoplasm. The role of the upper gastrointestinal series, endoscopy, endoscopic ultrasound, multidetector computed tomography (CT), magnetic resonance imaging, and positron emission tomography//CT in the diagnosis, treatment, staging, and follow-up of patients with gastric cancer is emphasized. The relative strengths and weaknesses of these diagnostic examinations will be presented in context with the most recent epidemiologic, pathologic, and therapeutic concepts regarding this tumor.

Only by a well orchestrated team approach including epidemiologists, diagnostic radiologists, gastroenterologists, oncologic surgeons, radiation oncologists, and pathologists, coupled with a better understanding of the molecular genetics of gastric cancer, can we hope to successfully address this major global health problem.

Richard M. Gore, MD

1

Epidemiology of gastric cancer

Mark E. Lockhart and Cheri L. Canon

Introduction

Although the incidence and mortality rate of gastric cancer are declining in the United States and Great Britain (Figures 1.1 and 1.2), gastric carcinoma remains the fourth most common cancer in the world [1] and is second only to lung cancer in terms of worldwide cancer deaths (Figures 1.3 and 1.4). The development of gastric cancer is a multifactorial process, and many conditions influence the likelihood of occurrence. An understanding of the disease process in these patients is important for the assessment of risk and prognosis. In this chapter, the epidemiologic factors of gastric cancer, including its incidence, mortality, pathogenesis, and risk factors, are discussed.

Incidence and mortality

In developing countries, there is a high incidence of gastric cancer, and more than 990 000 cases occur worldwide each year based on 2008 statistics [2, 3]. However, in the United States, gastric cancer represents only approximately 1.5% of an estimated 1.44 million new cancer cases each year [4]. There were 22 000 new cases in the United States in 2008. Despite the decreasing incidence of gastric carcinoma from a previous rate of 35/100 000 cases in 1930 to 4/100 000 cases in 2003, it carries a relatively high mortality rate when compared to other cancers: 2.96 and 5.70/100 000 for women and men, respectively. Not only is the incidence higher in men, so trends the death rate [4]. However, the mortality rate of gastric cancer in the United States has decreased by 26% and 35% since 1990 in females and males, respectively [4].

Gastric cancer is more common in older populations, usually occurring in the seventh and eighth decades of life. The mean age at diagnosis was 67 years in one large

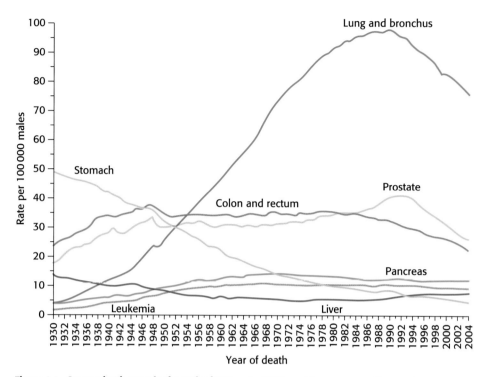

Figure 1.1. Cancer death rates in the United States. In 1930, gastric cancer was the most common cause of cancer-related deaths. By the twenty-first century, gastric cancer had become the seventh leading cause of cancer deaths in the United States.

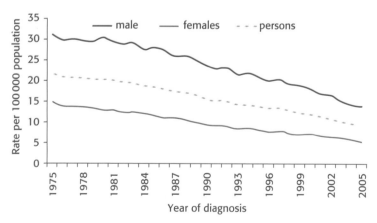

Figure 1.2. Age-standardized incidence rates of gastric cancer in Great Britain between 1975 and 2005.

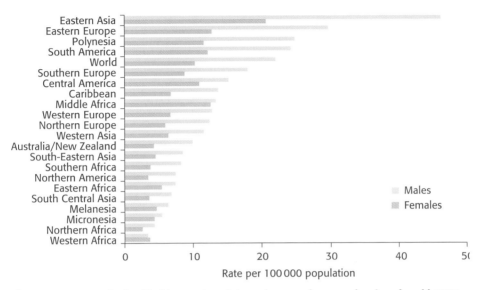

Figure 1.3. Age-standardized incidence rates of stomach cancer, by sex and region of world; 2008 estimates.

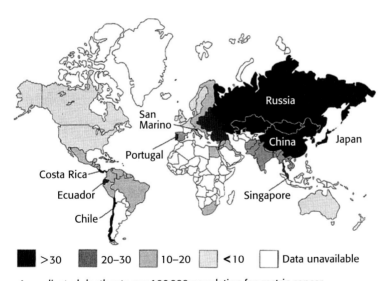

Age-adjusted death rate per 100 000 population for gastric cancer

Figure 1.4. Worldwide distribution of gastric cancer age-adjusted death rates. The highest incidences are found in the Far East, Russia, and Eastern Europe, and the lowest incidence rates are found in North America, Africa, the UK, Australia, and New Zealand. From Koh TJ and Wang TC. Tumors of the stomach. In Feldman M, Brandt LJ and Sleisenger MH eds., *Gastrointestinal and Liver Disease*, 7th edn. Philadelphia, PA: WB Saunders, 2002; pp. 822–59, figure 44.1, p. 830.

Table 1.1. Comparison of cardia and distal gastric adenocarcinoma

		Cardia adenocarcinoma	Distal adenocarcinoma
Change in incidence		++	–
Risk factors:	*H. pylori*	–	++
	Obesity	+	+/–
	Smoking	+	+
	Red meat	–	+
	Alcohol	?	?
	Low socioeconomic status	++	+
Prognosis		Worse	Better

series [5]. Although previously suspected, there is current uncertainty as to whether gastric cancer in young patients is associated with a worse clinical outcome [6].

Pathogenesis

Adenocarcinoma is the most common malignancy of the stomach, accounting for nearly 90% of gastric tumors [7]. Pathologically, there are two types of gastric adenocarcinoma based upon location: cardia, or proximal, and distal, non-cardia adenocarcinomas. These should be considered as separate entities because of differing epidemiologic relationships, associated risk factors, and prognosis [8] (Table 1.1). Historically, distal gastric carcinoma was the most common type. However, because the rate of cardia tumors continues to increase while that of distal gastric cancers decreases [9, 10], the incidence of proximal adenocarcinoma has surpassed that of distal cancers in recent years. This is an unfortunate change in the epidemiology of the disease since cancers of the gastric cardia generally have worse prognosis than distal gastric cancers [7, 10].

Histologically, gastric cancer is divided into two main types: well-differentiated, intestinal type, and undifferentiated, diffuse type [8]. The latter occurs in the setting of diffuse gastritis without atrophy. This histologic type is seen throughout the world, whereas the intestinal type occurs in areas with a high incidence of gastric cancer and follows a predictable stepwise progression of cancer development from metaplasia.

In 1994, the International Agency for Research on Cancer and The World Health Organization classified *Helicobacter pylori* (Figure 1.5) as a type I carcinogen, but

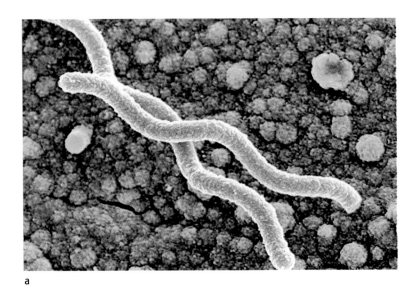

a

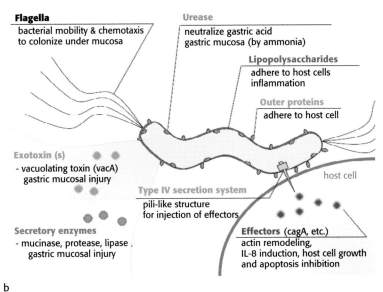

Flagella
bacterial mobility & chemotaxis
to colonize under mucosa

Urease
neutralize gastric acid
gastric mucosa (by ammonia)

Lipopolysaccharides
adhere to host cells
inflammation

Outer proteins
adhere to host cell

Exotoxin (s)
- vacuolating toxin (vacA)
  gastric mucosal injury

host cell

Type IV secretion system
pili-like structure
for injection of effectors

Secretory enzymes
- mucinase, protease, lipase
  gastric mucosal injury

Effectors (cagA, etc.)
actin remodeling,
IL-8 induction, host cell growth
and apoptosis inhibition

b

Figure 1.5. *Helicobacter pylori.* (a) Scanning electron micrograph image showing the wavy, thin, rod-shaped bacterium attached to the foveolar epithelium of the stomach. (b) Schematic diagram depicting the virulence factors of *Helicobacter pylori.* cagA, cytotoxin associated gene A.

the exact mechanism leading to gastric carcinoma is not clearly understood. The effects of *H. pylori* infection on gastric cancer appear multifactorial, involving host and environmental factors as well as differing bacterial strains. *H. pylori* is most closely associated with intestinal gastric cancers, which follow a stepwise pathway toward malignancy, similar to that in the colon. In the Correa model of gastric carcinogenesis, gastric inflammation leads to mucosal atrophy, metaplasia, dysplasia, and, ultimately, carcinoma [11]. Studies have shown that *H. pylori* infection is an independent risk factor for distal gastric cancer, with a 3- to 6-fold increased risk relative to those without the infection [12, 13, 14]. However, the great majority of infected individuals will never develop gastric neoplasia: approximately 40% of patients infected with *H. pylori* will develop gastric metaplasia but fewer than 1% will develop cancer [15].

Gastric atrophy also increases susceptibility of the cells to carcinogens. In patients with *H. pylori*, the presence of specific gene polymorphisms increases the risk of developing gastric carcinoma. Genes that encode tumor necrosis factor alpha (TNF-α), and interleukins IL-1, IL-8, and IL-10 have each been associated with higher cancer rates in the setting of *H. pylori* [16, 17]. While intestinal gastric cancer is strongly associated with chronic *H. pylori*, this strong link is not seen in diffuse gastric cancer. Diffuse or cardia gastric cancer, however, has been associated with other risk factors such as higher socioeconomic class [18], obesity [19, 20], and type A blood [21].

Risk factors

The risk factors for gastric cancer are protean and detailed in Table 1.2.

Ethnic and geographic factors

There is a higher incidence of gastric cancer in non-Caucasian populations. In the United States, the highest incidence is found in the Native American (21.6/100 000) and Asian (20/100 000) populations. Both race and sex affect the risk of disease development and subsequent mortality rate. The highest mortality rate based upon ethnic/sex combination is African-American males (12.4/100 000) [4]. However, there are similar overall 5-year survival rates among the different races.

The incidence of gastric carcinoma also varies dramatically by geographic location. In contrast to the American population, the societal burden of gastric cancer is much higher in Japan where it is the most common tumor type, accounting for approximately 19% of new tumor diagnoses based upon 2001 cancer registry data [22]. In Japanese men, the incidence rate is 116/100 000 [22]. A study by the American Cancer Society suggests that Japanese patients living within the United States who develop gastric cancer may even have differences in pathophysiology

Table 1.2. Risk factors for development of gastric cancer

Precursor conditions

Helicobacter pylori infection
Gastric adenomatous polyps
Chronic atrophic gastritis and intestinal metaplasia
Pernicious anemia
Partial gastrectomy for benign disease
Dietary
   Highly salted food
   Smoked foods, high fat or contaminated oil intake
   Low consumption of fruits and vegetables
Habits
   Smoking
   Consumption of sake or contaminated whiskey
Cultural
   Low socioeconomic status
Environmental
   Acidic or peaty soil
   High nitrate content in water
   Elevated lead or zinc in water
   Volcanic rock background
   Exposure to environmental talc
   Extensive use of nitrate fertilizers
   Urban residency
   Genetic
   Family history of gastric cancer
   Blood type A
   Hereditary non-polyposis colon cancer syndrome
   Familial adenomatous polyposis syndrome
   Peutz–Jeghers syndrome
   Li–Fraumeni syndrome
   Hyperplastic gastric polyposis
   Familial diffuse gastric carcinoma
Occupational
   Workers in mines and quarries
   Painters
   Fishermen
   Ceramic, clay, and stone workers
   Metal industry workers
   Agricultural workers
   Textile workers
   Printers and bookbinders

compared with their Caucasian counterparts. The percentage of cardia tumors in Japanese patients (11%) was less than half the percentage for the overall population in the study (28%) [5]. The study also showed that although gastric cancer is still more common in Japanese men than women, there was a smaller difference in the male-to-female ratio for Japanese patients compared with other Americans.

The rate of gastric cancer in other Asian countries such as Korea and China is also high. It is interesting to note that in similar parts of the world, incidence rates of gastric cancer can vary significantly. For example, within the European Union the highest mortality rate is found in Iceland and the lowest mortality rate is in Poland [23]. The mortality differs by the severity of disease at the time of diagnosis, and there is generally delayed diagnosis in Western populations as compared to in Japan. Still, there has been a long-term worldwide decrease in both the incidence and mortality associated with gastric cancer [24].

Genetics

There are a variety of genes that increase the risk of gastric cancer that are detailed in Table 1.3 and Figure 1.6. Specific genes such as MCC, APC, and p53 tumor suppressor genes have been identified in a large percentage of gastric cancers [25]. Several studies have identified E-cadherin, a calcium-dependent adhesion molecule that is responsible for cellular binding to adjacent cells, as an important component in the gastric carcinogenesis cascade [26, 27, 28]. Genetic susceptibility involves hereditary transmission of a single mutated CDH1 allele. If there is an acquired mutation of the second allele in the E-cadherin gene, then loss of intracellular adhesion leads to increased intracellular permeability [29]. A wide variety of mutations in this domain have been identified in gastric cancer families [30].

Multiple syndromes are associated with gastric carcinoma; most are associated with gastrointestinal polyp formation and have increased risk of cancer at other sites as well. These include familial adenomatous polyposis (FAP) and Cowden disease. The FAP genetic defect is located in the APC gene involved in the Wnt tumor-signaling pathway. This gene is located on chromosome 5q and involves development of different tumor types, including colonic and gastric cancers [31].

In FAP a significant proportion of adenomatous polyps in the stomach will develop into carcinoma. Hamartomatous polyps, such as are found in Peutz–Jeghers disease and juvenile polyposis, have exceedingly low malignant potential. However, patients with these syndromes tend also to have an increased incidence of adenomatous polyps, which do carry the risk of malignant transformation.

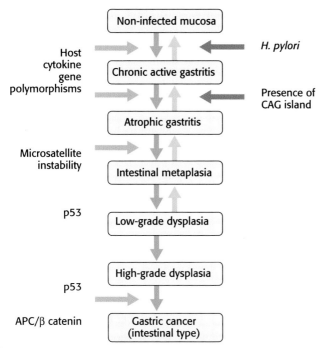

Figure 1.6. Proposed multistep pathway in the pathogenesis of gastric cancer. Infection with *Helicobacter pylori* is the common initiating event in most cases, and the presence of the *cag* pathogenicity island is associated with more severe disease. Host genetic polymorphisms, resulting in high production of interleukin-1β and tumor necrosis factor-α and low production of interleukin-10, contribute to gastric cancer risk. Accumulation of genetic defects within gastric lesions such as alterations in p53, microsatellite instability, and abnormalities in the adenomatous polyposis coli/β-catenin pathway may play a role in later steps. Gray arrows represent steps that are potentially reversible. (From Koh TJ, Wang TC: Tumors of the stomach. In Feldman M, Brandt LJ and Sleisenger MH eds., *Gastrointestinal and Liver Disease*, 7th edn. Philadelphia, PA: WB Saunders, 2002; pp. 822–59, Figure 44–4, p. 832.)

Hereditary diffuse gastric carcinoma is an autosomal dominant trait on chromosome 16p22 and has an associated 67%–83% lifetime risk of gastric carcinoma [32]. Families are identified if there are two first- or second-degree relatives who develop gastric cancer before age 50 or if there are three such relatives regardless of age. Due to the high risk of malignancy, genetic screening of patients' families is recommended if a patient is diagnosed with diffuse cancer before age 35, if the patient is diagnosed with gastric and breast carcinoma, or if family members have both diffuse gastric cancer and breast cancer [29].

In the absence of a defined familial syndrome, increased risk of gastric cancer is present in relatives of patients with breast cancer [33]. Also, the Li–Fraumeni

Table 1.3. Genetic alterations in gastric carcinomas and their relative frequency

Genes and alterations	Well-differentiated adenocarcinoma	Poorly differentiated adenocarcinoma
Telomerase activity	+++	+++
CD44 (abnormal transcript)	+++	+++
TGFA (overexpression)	++	++
DNA repair error	++	++
TP53 (LOH, mutation)	++	++
Beta catenin (mutation)	+	++
TP16 (reduced expression)	++	+
c-met (amplification)	+	++
VEGF (overexpression)	++	+
EGF (overexpression)	++	+
EGFR (overexpression)	++	+
APC (LOH, mutation)	++	+
DCC (LOH)	++	
BCL2 (LOH)	++	
E-cadherin/CDH1 gene		++
K-ras mutation	+	+
Cyclin E (amplification)	+	+
c-erbB-2 (amplification)	+	

The number of crosses defines the relative frequency, from + (infrequent) to +++ (very common genetic alteration); APC, adenomatous polyposis coli; EGF, epidermal growth factor; EGFR, EGF receptor; LOH, loss of heterozygosity; VEGF, vascular endothelial growth factor.

syndrome has an increased risk of breast and gastric cancer in addition to more commonly seen melanoma, leukemia, brain tumors, and sarcomas. The syndrome is autosomal dominant in inheritance and demonstrates high penetrance in the cancer predisposition. This cancer risk is associated with mutations involving tumor suppressor genes, specifically germline TP53 mutations [34].

Hereditary non-polyposis colorectal cancer (HNPCC, Lynch syndrome II) is a risk factor for stomach cancer. In nearly one-quarter of these patients with gastric cancer, chromosomal mutations result in microsatellite instability [35]. In this syndrome, there is an approximately 4-fold increase in stomach cancer relative to the general population [36]. The disease is transmitted in an autosomal dominant pattern and has a high degree of penetrance [37]. Patients with Lynch syndrome II more typically present with early onset of colorectal cancer, and patients are also at increased risk of uterine carcinoma [38].

In the absence of a known genetic syndrome, first-degree relatives of a patient with gastric cancer have a 2- to 3-fold higher risk of developing this neoplasm compared to the general population [39, 40]. In one study, the risk of gastric cancer for first-degree relatives was higher in patients with the diffuse form of gastric cancer [41]. In another endoscopic series of 270 first-degree relatives of gastric cancer patients 59% were *H. pylori* positive, and 30% had gastric mucosal metaplasia [42].

Environmental and behavioral factors

There are many environmental and behavioral factors that affect the development of gastric carcinoma (Table 1.2). Smoking is now considered a significant contributor. A meta-analysis in 1997 revealed a 44% increase in risk for gastric cancer for current and ex-smokers [43]. In a second more comprehensive meta-analysis in 2007, this increase in risk was reported as 60% for men and 20% for women [44]. In a population-based case control study, exposure to smoking at any time during the patient's life had a population-attributable risk of 18% and 45% for the development of both non-cardia and cardia gastric carcinomas, respectively [45]. The increase in cancer affects both cardia and non-cardia tumor types, with greater impact on female smokers [20]. Furthermore, smokers with chronic atrophic gastritis from *H. pylori* infection have increased rates of mucosal metaplasia and dysplasia relative to non-smokers [46, 47].

Unlike tobacco exposure, alcohol consumption has not been consistently shown to be associated with gastric cancer [20, 48, 49, 50, 51, 52]. Alcohol, however, has been identified as a risk factor for disease progression [53], and the combined effect of alcohol and smoking increases the risk of non-cardia gastric cancer 5-fold [50].

Diets with high amounts of fresh vegetables and fruit have been shown to have a protective association with gastric cancer [54, 55, 56, 57]. Study results evaluating the impact of a meat diet on the incidence of gastric cancer have had conflicting results. Two cohort studies found little or no association between total meat consumption and gastric cancer [58, 59]. Consumption of high levels of salt and processed meat has been shown to be positively associated with gastric cancer in some studies [54, 55, 56, 59, 60, 61], and no association has been shown in others [58, 62]. Yet all of these studies were performed outside of the United States, and, importantly, did not discriminate among cardia and non-cardia gastric cancer types.

In a more recent study performed in Canada, a Western diet of soft drinks, processed meats, refined grains, and sugars was associated with an increased risk of gastric adenocarcinoma for both men and women, while a "prudent" diet of fresh fruits and vegetables and fish demonstrated a one-third reduction in gastric cancer risk for women but not men [63]. In a European cohort study of 521 457 men and women, total meat intake, including fresh and processed red meat and poultry, was associated with an increased risk of non-cardia cancer, and an even higher risk for those with chronic *H. pylori* infection [64]. There was no association between diet and cancers of the cardia.

The method of meat preparation and cooking may also play a role in the development of gastric cancer. Heterocyclic amines (HAs), known mutagens and carcinogens, are produced when animal muscle is exposed to extreme heat. It is known that HAs are produced at increased levels with higher cooking temperatures. In a population-based case control interview study, not only was an increased risk for gastric cancer identified in those with a high intake of red meat, including processed meat, but also the risk was increased with increasing doneness of the meat [65]. There was a 3.2-fold increased risk of gastric cancer for those consuming well-done beef versus rare or medium-rare beef.

Nitrates present in foods, specifically *N*-nitroso compounds, have long been a suspected risk factor for stomach cancer [66]. Salted foods have been shown to increase the carcinogenic effects of nitrates in rats [67]. Nitrites represent a 41% population-adjusted risk for non-cardia gastric carcinoma [45]. In recent years there have been significant decreases in nitrite and nitrate levels in the diets of industrialized countries, which may be an important factor contributing to the lower gastric cancer rates observed in these areas [24].

Nitroso compounds may be encountered from exogenous sources as well as within foods. Certain occupations have been associated with the development of gastric cancer, and many are those that have recurrent exposure to dust in the workplace. Epidemiologic studies suggest that workers in the coal, rubber, asphalt, and leather industries have increased risk for gastric cancer. Rubber, metal, leather, and agriculture industries have increased exposure to *N*-nitrosamines [68]. Population studies in multiple countries have shown increased risk in occupations where workers are exposed to dust [69, 70].

Obese patients have an increased risk for cardia type gastric cancer [19, 20]. A large prospective cohort study revealed a body-mass-index- (BMI-) dependent increased risk of cardia gastric cancer in overweight (incidence rate ratio 1.32) and obese (2.73) subjects [19]. A similar association was demonstrated in two of three studies in a recent meta-analysis [71]. No association with height has been proven [19].

Pharmacologic factors can also have an impact on the incidence of gastric cancer. In one study, the use of aspirin or non-steroidal anti-inflammatory drugs was associated with approximately 50% decreased risk of non-cardia gastric adenocarcinomas [72]. Similar results were also reported after a prospective, nested case control study of over 2 million persons in the General Practitioners Database [73]. It has been hypothesized that long-term use of proton pump inhibitors (PPIs) could lead to carcinoid tumor or adenocarcinoma formation, but this has not proven to be true in current studies [74]. PPIs lead to a reduced acid state in the stomach, which, in turn, results in increased gastrin secretion. Carcinoids in this pathophysiologic scenario occur in Zollinger–Ellison syndrome (see "Carcinoid" below).

Pernicious anemia is another documented risk factor for gastric carcinoma. Pernicious anemia is a deficiency of intrinsic factor production by cells in the stomach that results in vitamin B12 deficiency. The long-term presence of gastric atrophy due to the pernicious anemia increases the incidence of gastric carcinoma. The population risk is small compared to that posed by other risk factors such as *H. pylori* infection.

Patients who have had gastric surgery for benign disease are also at 2–4 times increased risk for gastric cancer. This association may result from decreased acid production in the gastric remnant and chronic inflammation due to reflux of bile into the gastric remnant. In one study, the increased risk did not develop until approximately 20 years after the surgery [75]. Another study showed a nearly 2-fold risk of gastric cancer developing much sooner after surgery in men [76].

High-dose radiation exposure is an uncommon risk factor for gastric cancer found primarily in survivors of atomic bomb radiation in World War II [77].

A protective effect of vitamin C or beta-carotene has been previously associated with decreased gastric cancer rates. In a randomized, controlled chemoprevention trial, anti-*H. pylori* treatment, supplementation with ascorbic acid, and supplementation with beta-carotene were each associated with a significant regression of precancerous lesions in the setting of atrophic gastritis [78]. In a recent meta-analysis, antioxidants were found to have a protective role against esophageal cancer, and beta-carotene was found to be protective against cardia gastric cancer (odds ratio, OR, 0.57). In that study, vitamins C and E were not conclusively shown to reduce development of cardia gastric cancer [79].

Clearly, there are multiple factors that play a role in the development of gastric cancer, and, since cardia and non-cardia cancers have a different pathogenesis, their risk factors are very different. For cardia gastric cancers, smoking and elevated BMI were found to contribute 56.2% of the total cancer risk [45]. For non-cardia gastric cancers, smoking, history of gastric ulcers, elevated nitrite intake, and *H. pylori* infection combined to represent 59% of the cancer risk [45].

Lymphoma

Like gastric carcinoma, chronic *H. pylori* infection is the main risk factor for mucosa-associated lymphoid tissue (MALT) lymphoma, the most common lymphoma of the stomach [80]. In the absence of risk factors, lymphoma is not a common tumor of the stomach, which does not normally contain lymphoid tissue. Chronic inflammation leads to T-cell-mediated inflammation and lymphoid follicles, seen in 30% of those infected [80]. Treatment of the infection leads to remission in the majority of cases [81, 82]. However, some 20% of cases may require additional chemotherapy or surgery. These patients tend to have a more advanced lymphoma or a defined chromosomal translocation [83].

Gastrointestinal stromal tumor

Gastrointestinal stromal tumor (GIST) is a neoplasm that arises in the smooth muscle pacemaker cells of Cajal. It is pathologically identified by a tyrosine kinase membrane receptor, c-kit protein (CD 177 antigen). Most (66%) occur in the stomach and gastric GISTs have a lower malignant potential than tumors found elsewhere in the GI tract [84]. Like gastric carcinoma, GISTs may be associated with syndromes, but there is no overlap of the syndromes between the two cancer types. Syndromes associated with GIST include neurofibromatosis type I (von Recklinghausen disease), Carney triad, and familial GIST syndrome. Carney triad includes pulmonary chondroma and paraganglioma with gastric GIST.

Carcinoid

Carcinoid tumors are rare tumors of neuroendocrine cells that can arise in the GI tract or bronchial tree. All carcinoids are considered to have malignant potential [85] and are typically slow-growing. They most commonly occur in the small bowel, but the incidence of gastric carcinoid is increasing [86]. Only approximately 3% of carcinoids occur in the stomach [87]. Tumor location and patient age are the main predictors of pathologic behavior. Patients greater than 60 years of age have a poorer prognosis. Gastric carcinoids are less common in African-Americans than Caucasians [87].

There are groupings of gastric carcinoid tumors based upon clinical factors and prognosis. Type I is the most common form and usually represents benign disease. These carcinoids occur in the setting of autoimmune-mediated atrophic gastritis, where there is reduced gastric acid secretion by the decreased number of parietal cells. This leads to compensatory increased G-cell production of gastrin, resulting in hyperplasia of the enterochromaffin cells. Type I carcinoids are usually small, multiple, and located in the fundus. Unlike gastric carcinoma, they are more common in women (2.5:1). Patients have a mean age of 63 years at presentation [88]. Type II carcinoid occurs in the setting of multiple endocrine neoplasia (MEN) type I, which includes gastrinoma leading to Zollinger–Ellison syndrome, parathyroid hyperplasia, and pituitary and adrenal adenomas. Carcinoids in the setting of MEN I have a higher likelihood of malignancy than do type I tumors but, like type I tumors, they are often multiple in location. Patients with type II carcinoid are slightly younger than those with type I, with a mean age of 50 years, and there is no difference in incidence among men and women [88]. Type III carcinoids are sporadic, large, and usually aggressive. These carcinoids are more common in men, with a mean age of onset of 55 years [88].

Conclusion

In summary, gastric adenocarcinoma is an example of mixed success in the war against cancer. Since the 1970s, the overall incidence of gastric cancer has decreased. However, the more aggressive type makes up a larger percentage of all gastric cancers discovered. Many risk factors influence gastric cancer risk, i.e., genetic, life style, and environmental. An understanding of the epidemiology and risk factors may help in the diagnosis and determination of prognosis of this deadly worldwide disease [89].

REFERENCES

1. Brenner H, Rothenbacher D, and Arndt V. Epidemiology of stomach cancer. *Methods Mol Biol* 2009; **472**: 467–77.
2. de Vries AC and Kuipers EJ. Epidemiology of premalignant gastric lesions: implications for the development of screening and surveillance strategies. *Helicobacter* 2007; **12** Suppl 2: 22–31.
3. Katanoda K and Yako-Suketomo H. Comparison of time trends in stomach cancer incidence (1973–2002) in Asia, from cancer incidence in five continents, vols IV–IX. *Jpn J Clin Oncol* 2009; **39**(1): 71–2.

4. Jemal A, Siegel R, Ward E *et al.* Cancer statistics, 2008. *CA Cancer J Clin* 2009; **59**: 71–96.

5. Hundahl SA, Phillips JL, and Menck HR. The National Cancer Data Base Report on poor survival of U.S. gastric carcinoma patients treated with gastrectomy: Fifth Edition American Joint Committee on Cancer staging, proximal disease, and the "different disease" hypothesis. *Cancer* 2000; **88**(4): 921–32.

6. Lai JF, Kim S, Li C *et al.* Clinicopathologic characteristics and prognosis for young gastric adenocarcinoma patients after curative resection. *Ann Surg Oncol* 2008; **15**(5): 1464–9.

7. Fuchs CS and Mayer RJ. Gastric carcinoma. *N Engl J Med* 1995; **333**(1): 32–41.

8. Lauren P. The two histological main types of gastric carcinoma: diffuse and so-called intestinal-type carcinoma. An attempt at a histo-clinical classification. *Acta Pathol Microbiol Scand* 1965; **64**: 31–49.

9. He YT, Hou J, Chen ZF *et al.* Trends in incidence of esophageal and gastric cardia cancer in high-risk areas in China. *Eur J Cancer Prev* 2008; **17**(2): 71–6.

10. Maeda H, Okabayashi T, Nishimori I *et al.* Clinicopathologic features of adenocarcinoma at the gastric cardia: is it different from distal cancer of the stomach? *J Am Coll Surg* 2008; **206**(2): 306–10.

11. Correa P. Human gastric carcinogenesis: a multistep and multifactorial process – First American Cancer Society Award lecture on cancer epidemiology and prevention. *Cancer Res* 1992; **52**(24): 6735–40.

12. *Helicobacter* and Cancer Collaborative Group. Gastric cancer and *Helicobacter pylori*: a combined analysis of 12 case control studies nested within prospective cohorts. *Gut* 2001; **49**(3): 347–53.

13. Forman D, Newell DG, Fullerton F *et al.* Association between infection with *Helicobacter pylori* and risk of gastric cancer: evidence from a prospective investigation. *Br Med J* 1991; **302**(6788): 1302–5.

14. Parsonnet J, Friedman GD, Vandersteen DP *et al. Helicobacter pylori* infection and the risk of gastric carcinoma. *N Engl J Med* 1991; **325**(16): 1127–31.

15. Kuipers EJ. Review article: exploring the link between *Helicobacter pylori* and gastric cancer. *Aliment Pharmacol Ther* 1999; **13** Suppl 1: 3–11.

16. El-Omar EM, Carrington M, Chow WH *et al.* Interleukin-1 polymorphisms associated with increased risk of gastric cancer. *Nature* 2000; **404**(6776): 398–402.

17. Rad R, Dossumbekova A, Neu B *et al.* Cytokine gene polymorphisms influence mucosal cytokine expression, gastric inflammation, and host specific colonisation during *Helicobacter pylori* infection. *Gut* 2004; **53**(8): 1082–9.

18. Powell J and McConkey CC. Increasing incidence of adenocarcinoma of the gastric cardia and adjacent sites. *Br J Cancer* 1990; **62**(3): 440–3.

19. Merry AH, Schouten LJ, Goldbohm RA, and van den Brandt PA. Body mass index, height and risk of adenocarcinoma of the oesophagus and gastric cardia: a prospective cohort study. *Gut* 2007; **56**(11): 1503–11.

20. Lindblad M, Rodriguez LA, and Lagergren J. Body mass, tobacco and alcohol and risk of esophageal, gastric cardia, and gastric non-cardia adenocarcinoma among men and women in a nested case-control study. *Cancer Causes Control* 2005; **16**(3): 285–94.

21. Haenszel W, Correa P, Cuello C *et al.* Gastric cancer in Colombia. II. Case-control epidemiologic study of precursor lesions. *J Natl Cancer Inst* 1976; **57**(5): 1021–6.

22. Marugame T, Matsuda T, Kamo K, Katanoda K, Ajiki W, and Sobue T. Cancer incidence and incidence rates in Japan in 2001 based on the data from 10 population-based cancer registries. *Jpn J Clin Oncol* 2007; **37**(11): 884–91.

23. Coleman MP, Gatta G, Verdecchia A *et al.* EUROCARE-3 summary: cancer survival in Europe at the end of the 20th century. *Ann Oncol* 2003; **14** Suppl 5: v128–v49.

24. Howson CP, Hiyama T, and Wynder EL. The decline in gastric cancer: epidemiology of an unplanned triumph. *Epidemiol Rev* 1986; **8**: 1–27.

25. Rhyu MG, Park WS, Jung YJ, Choi SW, and Meltzer SJ. Allelic deletions of MCC/APC and p53 are frequent late events in human gastric carcinogenesis. *Gastroenterology* 1994; **106**(6): 1584–8.

26. Ilyas M and Tomlinson IP. The interactions of APC, E-cadherin and beta-catenin in tumour development and progression. *J Pathol* 1997; **182**(2): 128–37.

27. Brooks-Wilson AR, Kaurah P, Suriano G *et al.* Germline E-cadherin mutations in hereditary diffuse gastric cancer: assessment of 42 new families and review of genetic screening criteria. *J Med Genet* 2004; **41**(7): 508–17.

28. Guilford P, Hopkins J, Harraway J *et al.* E-cadherin germline mutations in familial gastric cancer. *Nature* 1998; **392**(6674): 402–5.

29. Robertson EV and Jankowski JA. Genetics of gastroesophageal cancer: paradigms, paradoxes, and prognostic utility. *Am J Gastroenterol* 2008; **103**(2): 443–9.

30. Oliveira C, Seruca R, and Carneiro F. Genetics, pathology, and clinics of familial gastric cancer. *Int J Surg Pathol* 2006; **14**(1): 21–33.

31. McKie AB, Filipe MI and Lemoine NR. Abnormalities affecting the APC and MCC tumour suppressor gene loci on chromosome 5q occur frequently in gastric cancer but not in pancreatic cancer. *Int J Cancer* 1993; **55**(4): 598–603.

32. Pharoah PD, Guilford P, and Caldas C. Incidence of gastric cancer and breast cancer in CDH1 (E-cadherin) mutation carriers from hereditary diffuse gastric cancer families. *Gastroenterology* 2001; **121**(6): 1348–53.

33. Burki N, Gencik A, Torhorst JK, Weber W, and Muller H. Familial and histological analyses of 138 breast cancer patients. *Breast Cancer Res Treat* 1987; **10**(2): 159–67.

34. Nichols KE, Malkin D, Garber JE, Fraumeni JFJ, and Li FP. Germ-line p53 mutations predispose to a wide spectrum of early-onset cancers. *Cancer Epidemiol Biomarkers Prev* 2001; **10**(2): 83–7.

35. Keller G, Grimm V, Vogelsang H *et al.* Analysis for microsatellite instability and mutations of the DNA mismatch repair gene hMLH1 in familial gastric cancer. *Int J Cancer* 1996; **68**(5): 571–6.

36. Watson P and Lynch HT. Extracolonic cancer in hereditary nonpolyposis colorectal cancer. *Cancer* 1993; **71**(3): 677–85.

37. Lynch HT, Smyrk TC, Watson P *et al.* Genetics, natural history, tumor spectrum, and pathology of hereditary nonpolyposis colorectal cancer: an updated review. *Gastroenterology* 1993; **104**(5): 1535–49.

38. Lynch HT and Smyrk T. Hereditary nonpolyposis colorectal cancer (Lynch syndrome). An updated review. *Cancer* 1996; **78**(6): 1149–67.

39. Zanghieri G, Di Gregorio C, Sacchetti C *et al.* Familial occurrence of gastric cancer in the 2-year experience of a population-based registry. *Cancer* 1990; **66**(9): 2047–51.

40. La Vecchia C, Negri E, Franceschi S, and Gentile A. Family history and the risk of stomach and colorectal cancer. *Cancer* 1992; **70**(1): 50–5.

41. Palli D, Galli M, Caporaso NE *et al.* Family history and risk of stomach cancer in Italy. *Cancer Epidemiol Biomarkers Prev* 1994; **3**(1): 15–18.

42. Leung WK, Ng EK, Chan WY *et al.* Risk factors associated with the development of intestinal metaplasia in first-degree relatives of gastric cancer patients. *Cancer Epidemiol Biomarkers Prev* 2005; **14**(12): 2982–6.

43. Trédaniel J, Boffetta P, Buiatti E, Saracci R, and Hirsch A. Tobacco smoking and gastric cancer: review and meta-analysis. *Int J Cancer* 1997; **72**(4): 565–73.

44. Ladeiras-Lopes R, Pereira AK, Nogueira A *et al.* Smoking and gastric cancer: systematic review and meta-analysis of cohort studies. *Cancer Causes Control* 2008; **19**(7): 689–701.

45. Engel LS, Chow WH, Vaughan TL *et al.* Population attributable risks of esophageal and gastric cancers. *J Natl Cancer Inst* 2003; **95**(18): 1404–13.

46. Russo A, Maconi G, Spinelli P *et al.* Effect of lifestyle, smoking, and diet on development of intestinal metaplasia in *H. pylori*-positive subjects. *Am J Gastroenterol* 2001; **96**(5): 1402–8.

47. Kneller RW, You WC, Chang YS *et al.* Cigarette smoking and other risk factors for progression of precancerous stomach lesions. *J Natl Cancer Inst* 1992; **84**(16): 1261–6.

48. Ye W, Ekstrom AM, Hansson LE, Bergstrom R, and Nyren O. Tobacco, alcohol and the risk of gastric cancer by sub-site and histologic type. *Int J Cancer* 1999; **83**(2): 223–9.

49. Lagergren J, Bergstrom R, Lindgren A, and Nyren O. The role of tobacco, snuff and alcohol use in the aetiology of cancer of the oesophagus and gastric cardia. *Int J Cancer* 2000; **85**(3): 340–6.

50. Sjödahl K, Lu Y, Nilsen TI *et al.* Smoking and alcohol drinking in relation to risk of gastric cancer: a population-based, prospective cohort study. *Int J Cancer* 2007; **120**(1): 128–32.

51. World Cancer Research Fund and American Institute for Cancer Research. *Food, Nutrition and Prevention of Cancer: a Global Perspective.* Washington, DC: American Institute of Cancer Research, 1997.

52. Gammon MD, Schoenberg JB, Ahsan H *et al.* Tobacco, alcohol, and socioeconomic status and adenocarcinomas of the esophagus and gastric cardia. *J Natl Cancer Inst* 1997; **89**(17): 1277–84.

53. Leung WK, Lin SR, Ching JY *et al.* Factors predicting progression of gastric intestinal metaplasia: results of a randomised trial on *Helicobacter pylori* eradication. *Gut* 2004; **53**(9): 1244–9.

54. Graham S, Haughey B, Marshall J *et al.* Diet in the epidemiology of gastric cancer. *Nutr Cancer* 1990; **13**(1–2): 19–34.

55. Risch HA, Jain M, Choi NW *et al.* Dietary factors and the incidence of cancer of the stomach. *Am J Epidemiol* 1985; **122**(6): 947–59.

56. Buiatti E, Palli D, Decarli A *et al.* A case-control study of gastric cancer and diet in Italy. *Int J Cancer* 1989; **44**(4): 611–16.

57. Lunet N, Valbuena C, Carneiro F, Lopes C, and Barros H. Antioxidant vitamins and risk of gastric cancer: a case-control study in Portugal. *Nutr Cancer* 2006; **55**(1): 71–7.

58. Ito LS, Inoue M, Tajima K *et al.* Dietary factors and the risk of gastric cancer among Japanese women: a comparison between the differentiated and non-differentiated subtypes. *Ann Epidemiol* 2003; **13**(1): 24–31.

59. Ngoan LT, Mizoue T, Fujino Y, Tokui N, and Yoshimura T. Dietary factors and stomach cancer mortality. *Br J Cancer* 2002; **87**(1): 37–42.

60. van den Brandt PA, Botterweck AA, and Goldbohm RA. Salt intake, cured meat consumption, refrigerator use and stomach cancer incidence: a prospective cohort study (Netherlands). *Cancer Causes Control* 2003; **14**(5): 427–38.

61. Buiatti E, Palli D, Decarli A *et al.* A case-control study of gastric cancer and diet in Italy: II. Association with nutrients. *Int J Cancer* 1990; **45**(5): 896–901.

62. Galanis DJ, Kolonel LN, Lee J, and Nomura A. Intakes of selected foods and beverages and the incidence of gastric cancer among the Japanese residents of Hawaii: a prospective study. *Int J Epidemiol* 1998; **27**(2): 173–80.

63. Campbell PT, Sloan M, and Kreiger N. Dietary patterns and risk of incident gastric adenocarcinoma. *Am J Epidemiol* 2008; **167**(3): 295–304.

64. Gonzalez CA, Jakszyn P, Pera G *et al.* Meat intake and risk of stomach and esophageal adenocarcinoma within the European Prospective Investigation into Cancer and Nutrition (EPIC). *J Natl Cancer Inst* 2006; **98**(5): 345–54.

65. Ward MH, Sinha R, Heineman EF *et al.* Risk of adenocarcinoma of the stomach and esophagus with meat cooking method and doneness preference. *Int J Cancer* 1997; **71**(1): 14–19.

66. Mirvish SS. The etiology of gastric cancer. Intragastric nitrosamide formation and other theories. *J Natl Cancer Inst* 1983; **71**(3): 629–47.

67. Tsugane S and Sasazuki S. Diet and the risk of gastric cancer: review of epidemiological evidence. *Gastric Cancer* 2007; **10**(2): 75–83.

68. Raj A, Mayberry JF, and Podas T. Occupation and gastric cancer. *Postgrad Med J* 2003; **79**(931): 252–8.

69. Dockerty JD, Marshall S, Fraser J, and Pearce N. Stomach cancer in New Zealand: time trends, ethnic group differences and a cancer registry-based case-control study. *Int J Epidemiol* 1991; **20**(1): 45–53.

70. Kneller RW, Gao YT, McLaughlin JK *et al.* Occupational risk factors for gastric cancer in Shanghai, China. *Am J Ind Med* 1990; **18**(1): 69–78.

71. Kubo A and Corley DA. Body mass index and adenocarcinomas of the esophagus or gastric cardia: a systematic review and meta-analysis. *Cancer Epidemiol Biomarkers Prev* 2006; **15**(5): 872–8.

72. Farrow DC, Vaughan TL, Hansten PD *et al.* Use of aspirin and other nonsteroidal anti-inflammatory drugs and risk of esophageal and gastric cancer. *Cancer Epidemiol Biomarkers Prev* 1998; **7**(2): 97–102.

73. Lindblad M, Lagergren J, and Garcia Rodriguez LA. Nonsteroidal anti-inflammatory drugs and risk of esophageal and gastric cancer. *Cancer Epidemiol Biomarkers Prev* 2005; **14**(2): 444–50.

74. Laine L, Ahnen D, McClain C, Solcia E, and Walsh JH. Review article: potential gastrointestinal effects of long-term acid suppression with proton pump inhibitors. *Aliment Pharmacol Ther* 2000; **14**(6): 651–68.

75. Stalnikowicz R and Benbassat J. Risk of gastric cancer after gastric surgery for benign disorders. *Arch Intern Med* 1990; **150**(10): 2022–6.

76. Fisher SG, Davis F, Nelson R, Weber L, Goldberg J, and Haenszel W. A cohort study of stomach cancer risk in men after gastric surgery for benign disease. *J Natl Cancer Inst* 1993; **85**(16): 1303–10.

77. Sauvaget C, Lagarde F, Nagano J, Soda M, Koyama K, and Kodama K. Lifestyle factors, radiation and gastric cancer in atomic-bomb survivors (Japan). *Cancer Causes Control* 2005; **16**(7): 773–80.

78. Correa P, Fontham ET, Bravo JC *et al.* Chemoprevention of gastric dysplasia: randomized trial of antioxidant supplements and anti-*Helicobacter pylori* therapy. *J Natl Cancer Inst* 2000; **92**(23): 1881–8.

79. Kubo A and Corley DA. Meta-analysis of antioxidant intake and the risk of esophageal and gastric cardia adenocarcinoma. *Am J Gastroenterol* 2007; **102**(10): 2323–30.

80. Marshall BJ and Windsor HM. The relation of *Helicobacter pylori* to gastric adenocarcinoma and lymphoma: pathophysiology, epidemiology, screening, clinical presentation, treatment, and prevention. *Med Clin North Am* 2005; **89**(2): 313–44.

81. Stolte M, Bayerdörffer E, Morgner A *et al.* Helicobacter and gastric MALT lymphoma. *Gut* 2002; **50** Suppl 3: 19–24.

82. Fischbach W, Goebeler-Kolve ME, Dragosics B, Greiner A, and Stolte M. Long term outcome of patients with gastric marginal zone B cell lymphoma of mucosa associated lymphoid tissue (MALT) following exclusive *Helicobacter pylori* eradication therapy: experience from a large prospective series. *Gut* 2004; **53**(1): 34–7.

83. Liu H, Ruskon-Fourmestraux A, Lavergne-Slove A *et al.* Resistance of t(11;18) positive gastric mucosa-associated lymphoid tissue lymphoma to *Helicobacter pylori* eradication therapy. *Lancet* 2001; **357**(9249): 39–40.

84. Miettinen M and Lasota J. Gastrointestinal stromal tumors: review on morphology, molecular pathology, prognosis, and differential diagnosis. *Arch Pathol Lab Med* 2006; **130**(10): 1466–78.

85. Levy AD and Sobin LH. From the archives of the AFIP: gastrointestinal carcinoids: imaging features with clinicopathologic comparison. *Radiographics* 2007; **27**(1): 237–57.

86. Modlin IM, Lye KD, and Kidd M. A 5-decade analysis of 13,715 carcinoid tumors. *Cancer* 2003; **97**(4): 934–59.

87. Modlin IM and Sandor A. An analysis of 8305 cases of carcinoid tumors. *Cancer* 1997; **79**(4): 813–29.

88. Rindi G, Bordi C, Rappel S, La Rosa S, Stolte M, and Solcia E. Gastric carcinoids and neuroendocrine carcinomas: pathogenesis, pathology, and behavior. *World J Surg* 1996; **20**(2): 168–72.

89. Sun P, Xiang JB, and Chen ZY. Meta-analysis of adjuvant chemotherapy after radical surgery for advanced gastric cancer. *Br J Surg* 2009; **96**(1): 26–33.

2

Pathology of gastric cancer

Curtis R. Hall

Introduction

The stomach is an eccentric tubular organ between the esophagus and the duode-num that functions as a food capacitor and, using hydrochloric acid and pepsin secreted by cells within it, contributes to food digestion. Like other components of the gastrointestinal (GI) tract, the stomach includes several layers of tissue, the two most relevant to a discussion of gastric neoplasia being the mucosa and the muscularis propria. The mucosa is subject to inflammatory processes, a familiar-ity with which aids in the understanding of the genesis of neoplasms arising from that layer of tissue. Neoplastic pathology of the stomach has been well reviewed in depth in recent years [1, 2, 3]; the following will serve as a brief introduction to the gross and microscopic characteristics of gastric neoplasms and their precursors, with special consideration of features relevant to prognosis. Current genetics and molecular biology of these processes will also be considered.

Gross and microscopical anatomy

The wall of the stomach is formed by several layers of tissue (Figure 2.1) [4]. The mucosa is the innermost layer and is derived from the fetal endoderm. The charac-ter of the mucosa varies somewhat depending on its location within the stomach. The mucosa lining the gastric fundus and body is made up of densely packed test-tube-like units divided into two zones: the pit and the gland. The pit, populated by tall mucus cells, extends from the surface to the glandular compartment, which is lined almost exclusively by parietal and chief cells. Parietal cells are the source of acid and intrinsic factor. Chief cells are the source of pepsinogen.

As with all epithelial structures, the cells lining these units rest upon a thin col-lagenous basement membrane, which serves to support the epithelial structures

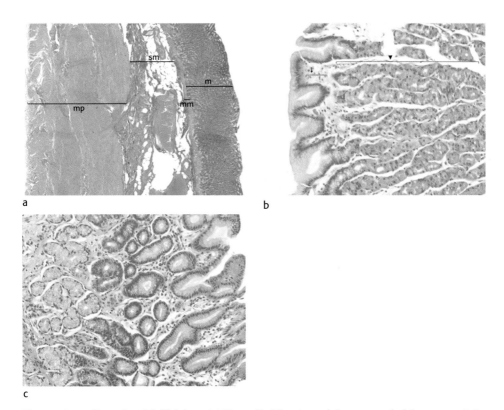

Figure 2.1a–c. Normal gastric histology. (a) The wall of the stomach is composed of the mucosa (m), muscularis mucosa (mm), submucosa (sm), and muscularis propria (mp). (b) Gastric body and fundus mucosa: the pit (arrow) communicates with the gland (arrowhead), which is populated by chief cells, parietal cells, and endocrine cells. The endocrine cells are difficult to identify in routine preparations. (c) Gastric antral mucosa: the epithelial structures consist almost entirely of pits; endocrine cells are present here as well.

and separate them from the lamina propria. Normal endocrine cells, involved in the regulation of acid secretion through the paracrinic secretion of histamine, sit between the basement membrane and the parietal and chief cells. In the gastric antrum, the test-tube-like structures are more widely spaced, shorter, and have abortive glandular zones. Endocrine cells are present here as well; 50% secrete gastrin. Of particular importance in the understanding of carcinogenesis is the fact that undifferentiated cells in the glandular compartment function as stem cells, which continuously regenerate to replace effete surface and pit epithelial cells as well as glandular cells. The lamina propria houses extracellular matrix proteins, small blood vessels, and nerve twigs. The muscularis mucosa is a thin layer of smooth muscle that separates the mucosa from the submucosa. The submucosa contains blood vessels, lymphatic channels, nerves, and extracellular matrix. The muscularis propria is a thick layer of smooth muscle with embedded neural elements including ganglion cells. The smooth muscle forming the muscularis propria wraps the stomach in three uniquely oriented bands.

Helicobacter pylori, gastritis, and peptic ulcer disease

The elucidation of the role the *Helicobacter pylori* bacterium plays in gastric pathology has been one of the major developments in medicine in the last 25 years [5, 6, 7]. *H. pylori* is a Gram-negative slow-growing, spiral bacillus which J. Robin Warren, a surgical pathologist in Perth, Australia, noticed as being consistently present in gastric mucosal biopsies demonstrating the long-recognized, characteristic inflammation he termed "active chronic gastritis." Later, *H. pylori* was demonstrated to be the cause of this gastritis, fulfilling Koch's hypothesis [8]. These gastric mucosal biopsies were taken from patients being evaluated for dyspepsia. Dyspepsia, a common complaint in Western countries [9], has been shown to be more firmly associated with peptic ulcer disease than simple active chronic gastritis [10]. In turn, peptic ulcer disease is strongly associated with *H. pylori*-induced gastritis [11].

An animal model, in which *H. pylori* induces peptic ulcer disease in Mongolian gerbils, has been developed to study this association [12, 13]. *Helicobacter*-associated gastritis is characterized by the presence of a population of lymphocytes in the lamina propria accompanied by infiltration of neutrophils between epithelial cells (Figure 2.2). In untreated cases, numerous *H. pylori* organisms are identifiable in the thick mucus that coats the surface of the mucosa. *H. pylori*-induced gastritis leads to gastric erosion and ulceration [12, 13, 14]. Approximately 80% of patients with peptic ulcers are infected with *H. pylori* [7]. In peptic ulcers, the mucosal surface is eroded and replaced with a mixed inflammatory infiltrate, fibrin, and granulation tissue. It has been shown that eradication of *H. pylori* organisms from the stomach promotes healing of peptic ulcers [6, 7]. In addition to ulceration, *H. pylori*-induced gastritis has been identified as the etiology of gastric atrophy and intestinal metaplasia [12, 13, 14], in which there is a loss of the acid-producing, glandular zone of the mucosa combined with replacement of surface epithelial cells by goblet cells reminiscent of those seen in the small intestinal epithelium. Gastric atrophy and intestinal metaplasia do not always supervene; a superficial chronic active gastritis may persist without such progression [7, 15]. In patients with *Helicobacter*-induced gastritis without atrophy and intestinal metaplasia, duodenal ulcer is more common than gastric ulcer.

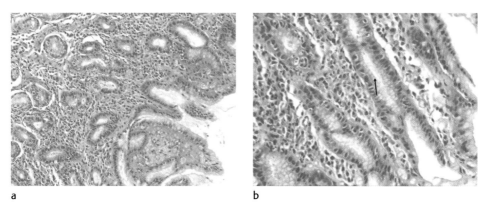

a   b

Figure 2.2a,b. *H. pylori*-induced gastritis. (a) Abnormal gastric mucosa with influx of multiple inflammatory cells. (b) Numerous *H. pylori* organisms are present in this field (arrow).

It should be noted that *H. pylori* is not the sole cause of gastritis [15], but it is the one most commonly associated with gastric neoplasia.

Gastric atrophy, intestinal metaplasia, and carcinogenesis

Severe gastric atrophy and its commonly associated intestinal metaplasia are closely associated with the intestinal type of gastric carcinoma (see further below) [16]. Ming further identified glandular dysplasia (cellular atypia without invasion) in association with this same type of gastric carcinoma (Figure 2.3) [17]. Severe gastric atrophy of the type associated with *H. pylori* ("multifocal atrophic gastritis") has been confirmed as a risk factor for gastric carcinoma in multiple studies. As a result, serum pepsinogen levels can be used as a screening tool for patients at high risk for gastric carcinoma [18]. It is hypothesized that there is a stepwise progression from *H. pylori*-induced gastritis, through atrophy, intestinal metaplasia, and dysplasia, to gastric carcinoma – the so-called "Correa sequence" [19]. This hypothesis, however, has been vigorously disputed [20]. Part of the difficulty in confirming this sequence lies in the task of differentiating glandular dysplasia (a non-invasive lesion) from early invasive carcinoma, a determination more subjective in the stomach than in other organs (e.g., uterus, cervix, breast, or even the colon). Reports of carcinoma developing in the Mongolian gerbil model have been disputed on this very point [21, 22, 23]. Nevertheless, studies have shown various molecular abnormalities in intestinal metaplasia (wherein microsatellite instability and *p53* and *APC* gene abnormalities have been identified) as well as other

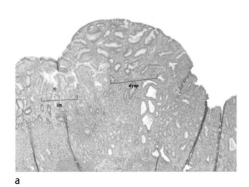
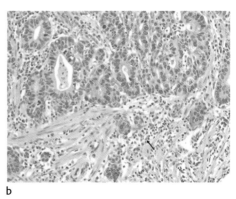

a   b

Figure 2.3a,b. The spectrum of intestinal metaplasia, dysplasia, and early carcinoma. (a) Intestinal metaplasia (im) and dysplastic epithelium (dysp) are visible on a background of gastritis. (b) Dysplastic glands with adjacent invasive carcinomatous glands (arrow).

putative pre-cancerous lesions [24], supporting the idea that the "Correa sequence" is correct.

The mechanism by which certain genes are silenced through methylation of promoter region CpG islands also appears to play a role in gastric carcinogenesis [25], as perhaps does the sonic hedgehog protein [26, 27]. Currently, the most widely accepted hypothesis for gastric carcinogenesis in sporadic cases is *H. pylori*-associated gastritis or the uncommon autoimmune gastritis that causes gastric atrophy. DNA lesions in the mucosal stem cells create genomic instability. Intestinal metaplasia may or may not be an intermediate step in this process. There is room in this hypothesis for the effects of other factors; for example, certain diets, prior gastric surgery, and gastric ulcers have all been shown to be associated with gastric carcinoma [3].

Gastric carcinoma

It has been estimated that there will have been 21 260 new cases of gastric cancer and 11 210 gastric cancer deaths in the United States in 2008 [28]. These numbers reflect a continuing downward trend in the incidence of gastric cancer since the 1940s. In 1930, the age-adjusted death rate for gastric cancer was approximately 49 per 100 000 men, while in 2003 this rate was approximately 5 per 100 000 men [28]. This trend indicates that the problems presented by gastric carcinoma are not new.

A widely referenced classification scheme for gastric carcinomas, based solely upon the gross features, was published in the German literature in the early twentieth

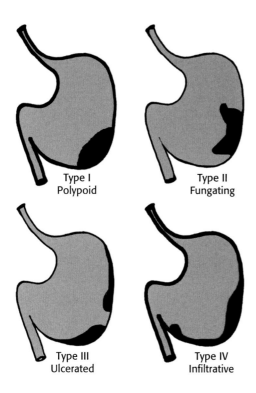

Figure 2.4. The Bormann gross classification system for gastric carcinoma.

Type I
Polypoid

Type II
Fungating

Type III
Ulcerated

Type IV
Infiltrative

century [1]. Bormann recognized four basic growth patterns for gastric carcinomas, and categorized them as follows (some tumors show a combination of these patterns): polypoid (type I), fungating (type II), ulcerated (type III), and diffusely infiltrative (type IV) (Figure 2.4). Type IV was also known as the linitis plastica growth pattern. It was recognized that a gastric ulcer may be benign or malignant. Gross features that have been associated with malignancy in gastric ulcers include irregular, heaped-up margins and a location on the greater curvature near the pylorus (Figure 2.5); in practice, confident differentiation of benign ulcers from malignant ulcers requires microscopic examination of biopsies in many cases [29].

On microscopic examination, gastric carcinomas show a variety of morphologies, and the World Health Organization (WHO) now recognizes several different microscopic types [1]. Gastric carcinoma may be segregated into two groups based on microscopic findings. In 1965, Pekka Lauren reported his experience, at the University of Turku in Finland, based on specimens taken from 1344 patients with gastric carcinoma from 1945 to 1964 [16]. Building on his own work and that of others, he found that he could segregate carcinomas of the stomach into two basic types, with a third group in which the tumors showed features of both

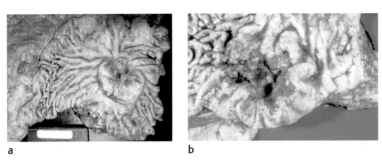

a   b

Figure 2.5a,b. Advanced gastric carcinoma: pathologic features. (a) Fungating gastric carcinoma (Bormann type II). (b) Malignant ulcer (Bormann type III).

of these two types. He grouped 53% of the tumors in his series as the "intestinal" type. Intestinal-type gastric carcinomas are usually characterized by the presence of gland-forming mitotically active columnar cells with enlarged, darkly staining (with hematoxylin) nuclei, with accumulation of mucin in the lumina of these malignant glands, and without much intracellular accumulation of mucin (Figure 2.6). He noted variations in this microscopic architecture: some specimens showed that the malignant cell primarily formed papillary structures while in others there was abundant mucin, forming pools ("colloid carcinoma"). The defining feature was the formation of relatively elaborate epithelial structures by cells exhibiting a high degree of cytological malignancy (nuclear enlargement, irregularity, and hyperchromasia). Interestingly, the malignant glands in these intestinal-type gastric carcinomas, as the name implies, were more reminiscent of the epithelial structures of the large intestine than of gastric glands. A consistent gross pathologic feature of this group of carcinomas is the presence of relatively well-defined tumors: 60% of these tumors were described as polypoid or fungating; only 15% were described as having a linitis plastica growth pattern.

Lauren found that 33% of the carcinomas in this series met the definition of the "diffuse" type. As compared to the cells in intestinal-type carcinomas, diffuse carcinoma cells were smaller, more uniform in overall shape and in nuclear size, and had less mitotic activity (Figure 2.7). Epithelial structures formed by these cells were more abortive, with only rare lumen formation. To the naked eye, diffuse carcinomas did not form well-defined masses in many cases, and microscopically showed extensive infiltration of the mucosa without associated ulceration. Thirty-one per cent of these tumors were described as polypoid or fungating; 43% were described as having a linitis plastica growth pattern.

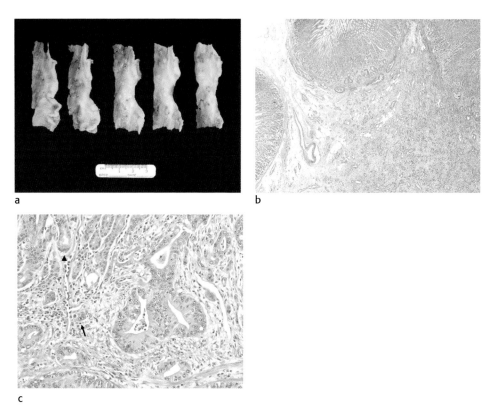

Figure 2.6a–c. Intestinal-type gastric carcinoma: pathologic features. (a) Note the relatively well-defined margin of this tumor on cross-section. (b) Low magnification view of intestinal-type carcinoma. (c) This image contrasts the nuclear features of malignant glands (arrow) with those of benign glands (arrowhead).

Lauren noted that these two types of gastric carcinoma tended to arise in different backgrounds. Intestinal-type carcinomas were seen more often (88% vs. 45%) in a background of gastritis and "profuse" intestinal metaplasia (37% vs. 7%) compared to diffuse carcinomas. There were demographic differences between the two tumor types as well. In patients with intestinal-type carcinoma, 65% were men and the average age was 55.4 years; in diffuse-type gastric carcinoma, 54% were men and the average age was 47.7 years.

Though there have been attempts to improve upon the Lauren classification, this system remains the most commonly encountered in the literature. Of note, the relationship between intestinal-type carcinomas and intestinal metaplasia was confirmed by Ming, with the additional finding that there was often glandular

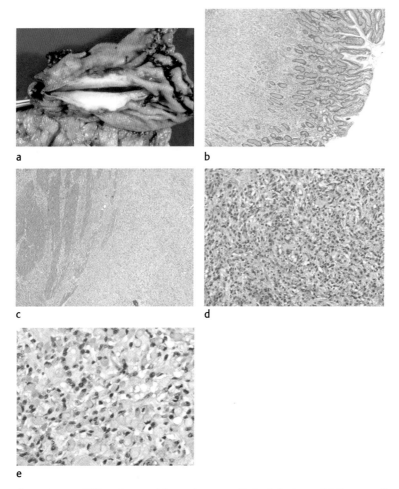

Figure 2.7a–e. Diffuse-type gastric carcinoma: pathologic features. (a) Cross-section of diffuse-type carcinoma: linitis plastica, Bormann type IV. (b) Tumor cells fill the lamina propria, leaving benign glands largely undisturbed. (c) Tumor cells infiltrate the muscularis propria. (d) In diffuse-type carcinoma, glandular structures are abortive. (e) In this field, many tumor cells have a signet-ring appearance.

dysplasia (cellular atypia) in the background of intestinal-type carcinomas, while this was "rare" in the background of diffuse-type carcinomas [17].

Compared with diffuse-type tumors, tumors of the intestinal type occur in an older age population, have a greater male:female ratio, and appear to arise in the milieu of gastritis/atrophy/intestinal metaplasia and epithelial dysplasia. Diffuse-type tumors usually arise in a background of a histologically normal stomach without precursor lesions. In view of the differences in these two types of tumor, it has been postulated that there are two pathways that lead to carcinoma in the stomach [25].

Tumors of the intestinal type are thought to arise through a stepwise progression, often starting with *H. pylori*-induced gastritis, which has been discussed. While there is a relationship between diffuse-type gastric carcinoma and *H. pylori*-induced gastritis (of the non-atrophic variety), no intermediate lesions are operative [25]. There is some molecular overlap between the two types of gastric carcinoma; for example, mutations in the tumor suppressor gene *TP53* are seen in both types of gastric carcinoma, as is silencing (by hypermethylation) of the mismatch repair gene *MGMT*. However, there are molecular defects unique to one or the other of these types of gastric carcinoma; abnormalities of *K-RAS*, *APC*, and *ERBB2* are confined to the intestinal type, for example. Defects in the *CDH1* gene are almost exclusive to diffuse-type carcinomas. The *CDH1* gene codes for the e-cadherin protein, which is important in cell–cell adhesion. Loss of expression of this protein correlates with loss of cohesion, leading to tumors that diffusely infiltrate as single or small groups of cells, often with intracellular accumulation of mucin giving a signet-ring appearance to the individual cells. This phenotype is mirrored by infiltrating lobular carcinoma of the breast.

In the familial syndrome hereditary diffuse gastric carcinoma (HDGC), diffuse gastric carcinoma and occasionally infiltrating lobular carcinoma of the breast develop in young adults [30]. Mutations in the *CDH1* gene have been characterized in many of these families. Individuals in these families are offered prophylactic gastrectomy [31]. Other familial syndromes in which there are increased rates of gastric carcinoma include familial adenomatous polyposis, Lynch syndrome, Li–Fraumeni syndrome, and Peutz–Jeghers syndrome [32].

There is evidence that carcinomas that arise in the gastric cardia are a heterogeneous group of neoplasms. One set has the same genesis as tumors of the more distal stomach and the other set is composed of tumors that are more closely related to adenocarcinomas of the distal esophagus, which are strongly associated with intestinal metaplasia (Barrett esophagus) [33, 34]. While the incidence of gastric carcinoma has been decreasing, the incidence of carcinomas of the cardia has been increasing for unknown reasons [34].

Regardless of its etiology, carcinoma of the gastric cardia is microscopically indistinguishable from carcinoma of the more distal stomach and should be assessed in the same manner. A separate issue is that group of tumors which straddle the gastro-esophageal junction, making it difficult to determine whether they are of esophageal or cardia origin.

While the Lauren classification system has been of great help in furthering the understanding of gastric carcinoma biology and pathogenesis, the most reliable predictor of outcome for gastric carcinoma has proven to be the staging systems that take into account the depth of tumor invasion, regional lymph node status, and the presence or absence of distant metastases (see Chapter 7) [35, 36]. The 5-year survival for patients with Stage IA gastric carcinoma is 78%; the 5-year survival for patients with Stage IV gastric carcinoma is 7% [35]. Obviously early detection and treatment lead to improved patient survival.

In Japan, where an endemically high rate of gastric carcinoma prompted the institution of a program of screening by upper endoscopy, experience with such early-stage gastric carcinomas has accrued. Tumors meeting the definition of "early gastric carcinoma" do not invade any deeper into the gastric wall than the submucosa. Tumors which invade into the muscularis propria or deeper are called "advanced gastric carcinoma." They may be amenable to endoscopic resection, as opposed to gastrectomy (see Chapter 3) [37]. A gross morphologic classification of early gastric carcinoma into five groups has been formulated (Figure 2.8) and is now used internationally [38].

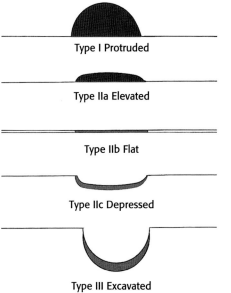

Type I Protruded

Type IIa Elevated

Type IIb Flat

Type IIc Depressed

Type III Excavated

Figure 2.8. The Japanese classification system for early gastric carcinoma.

Gastric lymphoma

Primary gastric lymphoma accounts for 7% of primary gastric neoplasms [39]. *H. pylori* infection is considered to be the ultimate cause of most primary gastric lymphomas. The normal stomach harbors few lymphocytes, but the inflammatory reaction to *H. pylori* induces lymphocytic migration into the gastric mucosa [40]. The arriving lymphocytes assemble into an organoid structure resembling a lymph node, with follicular, interfollicular, and intraepithelial populations of lymphocytes. Thus, this lymphocytic population assumes a relationship with the gastric mucosa much like that seen in the constitutive mucosa-associated lymphoid tissue (MALT) of other organs, including the terminal ileum and appendix. Through the proliferative effect of continuous antigenic stimulation, with acquisition of molecular defects [e.g., t(11;18)], a low-grade lymphoma may arise out of this *H. pylori*-induced gastric MALT. This neoplasm has a characteristic morphology and behavior common to lymphomas arising in other portions of the gut colloquially referred to as "MALTomas." These often indolent tumors, which have the more formal and descriptive designation of "low-grade B-cell lymphoma of extranodal marginal zone (MALT) type" [40], are composed of regular, relatively small lymphocytes with light-staining cytoplasm (Figure 2.9). Expansion of the lamina propria by these cells

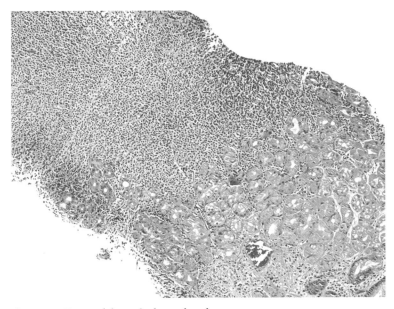

Figure 2.9. Extranodal marginal zone lymphoma.

is the key feature allowing differentiation from an intense *H. pylori*-induced gastritis [40]. Pathologists are encouraged to avoid being more definitive than the histologic findings warrant; the natural history of these tumors allows the luxury of waiting until the process declares itself morphologically. Once a diagnosis is established, there are several treatment options for these tumors, including eradication of *H. pylori*; gastric MALTomas will often respond to this measure [39].

Sixty per cent of primary gastric lymphomas are not the indolent, low-grade tumors described above but rather are aggressive, high-grade, diffuse, large B-cell lymphomas [39], in which the neoplastic cells are large, immature, proliferating lymphocytes (Figure 2.10). They may arise in a background of a MALToma or apparently de novo. These high-grade lymphomas often are tumor forming, may be associated with hematemesis or perforation, and can be difficult to distinguish from a poorly differentiated carcinoma both grossly and microscopically. Immunoperoxidase stains for lymphoid and epithelial markers are often diagnostic [39].

Gastric carcinoid and other neuroendocrine tumors

Gastritis, which plays such an important role in the genesis of gastric carcinoma and lymphoma, also potentiates the development of gastric carcinoid tumors. As in other organs, gastric carcinoid tumors are well-differentiated neoplasms of endocrine cells. With chronic atrophic gastritis, the loss of the acid-generating capacity of the gastric body and fundus causes loss of feedback control over the gastrin-secreting endocrine cells of the gastric antrum. Gastrin induces hyperplasia of the histamine-secreting endocrine cells of the gastric fundus and body. Gastric carcinoid tumors that develop as a result of this pathophysiologic scenario have been

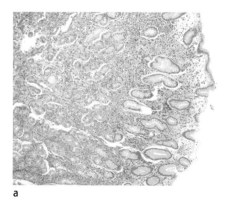
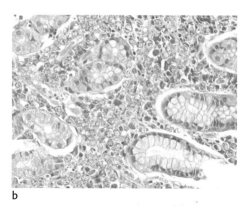

a   b

Figure 2.10a,b. Gastric diffuse large B-cell lymphoma. (a) Low magnification view. (b) Note the large nuclei which occupy most of each cell.

termed type I gastric carcinoids and comprise 80% of all these tumors [41]. Some 6% of gastric carcinoids are type II, in which the source of gastrin is a neoplasm of gastrin-secreting endocrine cells (usually located in the pancreas or small intestine) developing in patients with multiple endocrine neoplasia (MEN). Gastric carcinoids rarely develop in this Zollinger–Ellison scenario outside the MEN setting; presumably the molecular defect of MEN is a prerequisite [41, 42]. Finally, 14% of gastric carcinoids are type III, in which the tumors are sporadic, without a background gastrin-induced endocrine hyperplasia [41].

Whatever their pathogenesis, carcinoid tumors are mucosal-based nodules composed of uniform, polygonal cells with finely divided chromatin and small nucleoli, if present, that are small (Figure 2.11). Type III tumors may have more worrisome microscopic features, such as vesicular nuclei and mitotic activity [42]. Types I and II tumors are often multiple, with maximum dimensions uncommonly greater than 2 cm. Type I tumors tend to be small, with 77% measuring less than 1 cm in greatest dimension [41].

The sporadic (type III) tumors are most often single and tend to be larger, with 33% measuring larger than 2 cm in greatest dimension. Types I and II tumors are most often confined to the mucosa and behave benignly, while the sporadic tumors invariably

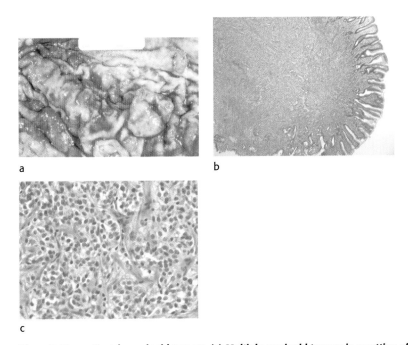

a

b

c

Figure 2.11a–c. Gastric carcinoid tumors. (a) Multiple carcinoid tumors in a setting of atrophic gastritis. (b) Low magnification view. (c) High magnification view shows round, regular nuclei with finely divided nuclear material and small nucleoli.

have spread beyond the mucosa, with a metastasis rate of 50%–70%, at presentation [41, 42]. As the behavior of carcinoid tumors cannot be predicted based on morphologic features or degree of local spread, no staging system has been developed.

As opposed to the histologically well-differentiated endocrine tumors described above, there is a small subset of poorly differentiated, overtly malignant mucosal-based gastric tumors whose endocrine differentiation is often only hinted at on routine microscopic examination. Confirmation of these tumors requires special studies such as immunohistochemistry and electron microscopy [41]. Of 12 tumors in this category, which have been termed poorly differentiated neuroendocrine carcinomas, 100% involved at least the muscularis propria and had metastasized, with 50% having metastasized to distant sites. Of 12 of these patients, 9 had died within a year [41].

Gastric stromal tumors

In the past, tumors arising in the muscularis propria of the stomach were considered to be neoplasms of smooth muscle such as leiomyomas and leiomyosarcomas. It is now understood that most tumors of the gastric muscularis propria are gastrointestinal stromal tumors (GISTs). GISTs may arise anywhere in the GI tract, but 60% occur in the stomach [43]. Gastric GISTs occur at a rate of 0.31 per 100 000 [44]. Mutations in either KIT or platelet-derived growth factor alpha (PDGFA), genes for two closely related tyrosine kinases, have been detected in more than 80% of GISTs [43]. These activating mutations lead to overexpression of the Kit receptor tyrosine kinase (CD117), making positivity for CD117 by the immunoperoxidase technique near-diagnostic for GISTs. This molecular defect renders them amenable to treatment with imatinib mesylate (Gleevec), a tyrosine kinase inhibitor.

Gastrointestinal stromal tumors have a varied morphology (Figure 2.12) [43]. On microscopic examination, some resemble smooth muscle tumors, some resemble peripheral nerve sheath tumors, and some have an idiosyncratic paucicellular character in which there are bland spindled cells in a collagenous background. GIST cells may have an epithelioid (polygonal) morphology, particularly in the stomach.

There is a continuum of possible outcomes for GISTs, from benign (no recurrence) to malignant (recurrence, metastasis, and death). GISTs are best placed on this continuum by assessing two parameters: tumor size and mitotic activity [43]. For gastric GISTs, tumors that are 2 cm or less in maximum dimension and show 5 (or fewer) mitotic figures per 50 high-powered fields (HPF) behave benignly, while 86% of tumors greater than 10 cm in maximum dimension and with mitotic rates greater than 5 per 50 HPF behave aggressively.

Other tumors

True leiomyomas, leiomyosarcomas, and benign and malignant peripheral nerve sheath tumors do occur in the stomach, albeit at a low rate. Malignant melanoma and infiltrating lobular carcinoma of the breast have a particular propensity to metastasize to the GI tract. Metastatic lobular carcinoma can be very difficult to differentiate from the diffuse type of primary gastric carcinoma.

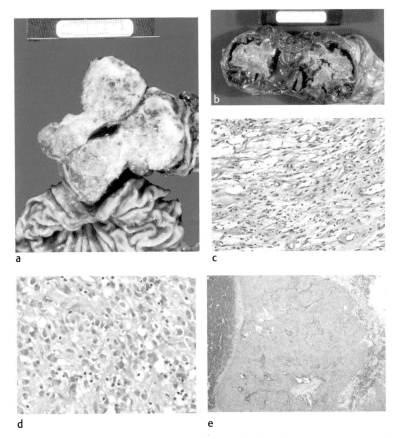

Figure 2.12a–i. Gastrointestinal stromal tumors (GIST): pathologic spectrum. (a) Gross specimen. (b) GIST with extensive necrosis. (c) Relatively paucicellular GIST with spindled and epithelioid cells. (d) Same tumor as in (c); here, the epithelioid cells dominate the field. (e) A more cellular GIST dominated by spindled cells.

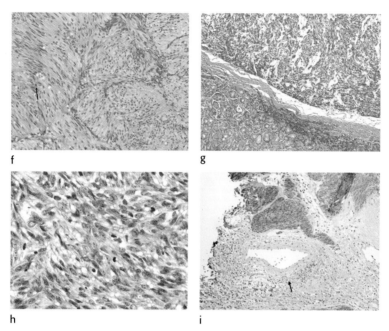

Figure 2.12. (Cont.) (f) Same tumor as in (e); in this field, the tumor cell nuclei arrange themselves in structures (Verocay bodies, arrow) reminiscent of those seen in peripheral nerve sheath tumors. (g) Highly cellular GIST; this large tumor has aggressive features. (h) Same tumor as in (g); note the mitotic figures. (i) GIST stained for CD117 by the immunoperoxidase technique; note the negative vascular smooth muscle cells (arrow).

Summary

Gastric carcinoma behaves as two distinct diseases. The intestinal type expands through the gastric wall whereas the diffuse type is primarily infiltrative. The intestinal (expansile) type of gastric cancer predominates in high-risk populations and for this reason has also been called the "epidemic type." Diffuse-type gastric cancer is less common in all countries and has been called the "endemic type." Intestinal-type cancer occurs most often in elderly men, is associated with a better survival, and is preceded by multifocal atrophic gastritis, typically due to *H. pylori* infection. Diffuse-type gastric cancers generally occur in women and individuals younger than age 50, have a poorer prognosis, and usually are not preceded by a histologically identifiable precursor lesion.

REFERENCES

1. Fenoglio-Preiser C, Munoz N, Carneiro F *et al*. Gastric cancer. In Hamilton SR and Aaltonen LA eds., *Pathology and Genetics: Tumours of the Digestive System*. Lyon, France: IARC Press, 2000; pp. 38–52.

2. Day DW, Jass JR, Price AB *et al. Morson and Dawson's Gastrointestinal Pathology*, 4th edn. Malden, MA: Blackwell Science, 2003; pp. 162–213.

3. Fenoglio-Preiser CM, Noffsinger AE, Stemmerman GN *et al.* The neoplastic stomach. In *Gastrointestinal Pathology: An Atlas and Text*, 3rd edn. Philadelphia, PA: Lippincott Williams & Wilkins, 2008; pp. 233–73.

4. Owen DA. Stomach. In Sternberg SS ed., *Histology for Pathologists*, 2nd edn. Philadelphia, PA: Lippincott-Raven, 1997; pp. 481–93.

5. Warren JR and Marshall B. Unidentified curved bacilli on gastric epithelium in active chronic gastritis. *Lancet* 1983; **1**: 1273–5.

6. Marshall B. *Helicobacter pylori*: 20 years on. *Clin Med* 2002; **2**: 147–52.

7. Atherton JC. The pathogenesis of *Helicobacter pylori*-induced gastro-duodenal diseases. *Annu Rev Pathol Mech Dis* 2006; **1**: 63–96.

8. Taylor DN and Blaser MJ. The epidemiology of *Helicobacter pylori* infection. *Epidemiol Rev* 1991; **13**: 42–59.

9. van Kerkhoven LAS, Eikandal T, Laheij RJF *et al.* Gastrointestinal symptoms are still common in a general Western population. *Neth J Med* 2008; **66**: 18–22.

10. Tahara T, Arisawa T, Shibata T *et al.* Association of endoscopic appearances with dyspeptic symptoms. *J Gastroenterol* 2008; **43**: 208–15.

11. Marshall BJ and Warren JR. Unidentified curved bacilli in the stomach of patients with gastritis and peptic ulceration. *Lancet* 1984; **1**: 1311–14.

12. Honda S, Fujioka T, Tokieda M *et al.* Gastric ulcer, atrophic gastritis and intestinal metaplasia caused by *Helicobacter pylori* infection in Mongolian gerbils. *Scand J Gastroenterol* 1998; **33**: 454–60.

13. Ikeno T, Ota H, Sugiyama A *et al. Helicobacter pylori*-induced chronic active gastritis, intestinal metaplasia, and gastric ulcer in Mongolian gerbils. *Am J Pathol* 1999; **154**: 951–60.

14. Zhang C, Yamada N, Wu Y-L *et al. Helicobacter pylori* infection, glandular atrophy and intestinal metaplasia in superficial gastritis, gastric erosion, erosive gastritis, gastric ulcer and early cancer. *World J Gastroenterol* 2005; **11**: 791–6.

15. Owen DA. Gastritis and carditis. *Mod Pathol* 2003; **16**: 325–41.

16. Lauren P. The two histological main types of gastric carcinoma: diffuse and so-called intestinal-type carcinoma. *Acta Pathol Microbiol Scand* 1965; **64**: 31–49.

17. Ming S-C. Gastric carcinoma: a pathobiological classification. *Cancer* 1977; **39**: 2475–85.

18. Ohata H, Kitauchi S, Yoshimura N *et al.* Progression of chronic atrophic gastritis associated with *Helicobacter pylori* infection increases risk of gastric cancer. *Int J Cancer* 2004; **109**: 138–43.

19. Correa P. Human gastric carcinogenesis: a multistep and multifactorial process. *Cancer Res* 1992; **52**: 6735–40.

20. Meining A, Morgner A, Miehlke S *et al.* Atrophy-metaplasia-dysplasia-carcinoma sequence in the stomach: a reality or merely an hypothesis? *Best Pract Res Clin Gastroenterol* 2001; **15**: 983–98.

21. Elfvin A, Bölin I, von Bothmer C *et al. Helicobacter pylori* induces gastritis and intestinal metaplasia but no gastric adenocarcinoma in Mongolian gerbils. *Scand J Gastroenterol* 2005; **40**: 1313–20.

22. Zheng Q, Chen XY, Shi Y *et al.* Development of adenocarcinoma in Mongolian gerbils after long-term infection with *Helicobacter pylori. J Gastroenterol Hepatol* 2004; **19**: 1192–8.

23. Watanabe T, Tada M, Nagai H *et al. Helicobacter pylori* infection induces gastric cancer in Mongolian gerbils. *Gastroenterology* 1998; **115**: 642–8.

24. Gologan A, Graham DY, and Sepulveda AR. Molecular markers in *Helicobacter pylori*-associated carcinogenesis. *Clin Lab Med* 2005; **25**: 197–222.

25. Vauhkonen M, Vauhkonen H, and Sipponen P. Pathology and molecular biology of gastric cancer. *Best Pract Res Clin Gastroenterol* 2006; **20**: 651–74.

26. Shiotani A, Iishi H, Uedo N *et al.* Evidence that loss of sonic hedgehog is an indicator of *Helicobacter pylori*-induced atrophic gastritis progressing to gastric cancer. *Am J Gastroenterol* 2005; **100**: 581–7.

27. Wang L-H, Choi Y-L, Hua X-Y *et al.* Increased expression of sonic hedgehog and altered methylation of its promoter region in gastric cancer and its related lesions. *Mod Pathol* 2006; **19**: 675–83.

28. Brenner H, Rothenbacher D, and Arndt V. Epidemiology of stomach cancer. *Methods Mol Biol* 2009; **472**: 467–77.

29. Adachi Y, Mori M, Tsuneyoshi M *et al.* Benign gastric ulcer grossly resembling a malignancy: a clinicopathological study of 20 resected cases. *J Clin Gastroenterol* 1993; **16**: 103–8.

30. Bacani JT, Soares M, Zwingerman R *et al.* CDH1/E-cadherin germline mutations in early-onset gastric cancer. *J Med Genet* 2006; **43**: 867–72.

31. Chung DC, Yoon SS, Lauwers GY *et al.* Case 22–2007: a woman with a family history of gastric and breast cancer. *New Engl J Med* 2007; **357**: 283–91.

32. Lynch HT, Grady W, Suriano G *et al.* Gastric cancer: new genetic developments. *J Surg Oncol* 2005; **90**: 114–33.

33. Derakhshan MH, Malekzadeh R, Watabe H *et al.* Combination of gastric atrophy, reflux symptoms and histological subtype indicates two distinct aetiologies of gastric cardia cancer. *Gut* 2008; **57**: 298–305.

34. McColl KEL. Cancer of the gastric cardia. *Best Pract Res Clin Gastroenterol* 2006; **20**: 687–96.

35. Greene FL, Page DL, Fleming ID *et al.* eds. Stomach. In *AJCC Cancer Staging Manual*, 6th edn. New York, NY: Springer, 2002; pp. 99–103.

36. Maruyama K. The most important prognostic factors for gastric cancer patients: a study using univariate and multivariate analyses. *Scand J Gastroenterol* 1987; **22** (S133): 63–8.

37. Okabayashi T, Kobayashi M, Nishimori I *et al.* Clinicopathological features and medical management of early gastric cancer. *Am J Surg* 2008; **195**: 229–32.

38. Ohta H, Noguchi Y, Takagi K *et al.* Early gastric carcinoma with special reference to macroscopic classification. *Cancer* 1987; **60**: 1099–106.

39. Morgner A, Schmelz R, Thiede C *et al.* Therapy of gastric mucosa associated lymphoid tissue lymphoma. *World J Gastroenterol* 2007; **13**: 3554–66.

40. Banks PM. Gastrointestinal lymphoproliferative disorders. *Histopathology* 2007; **50**: 42–54.

41. Rindi G, Bordi C, Rappel S *et al.* Gastric carcinoids and neuroendocrine carcinoma: pathogenesis, pathology, and behavior. *World J Surg* 1996; **20**: 168–72.

42. Levy AD and Sobin LH. Gastrointestinal carcinoids: imaging features with clinicopathologic comparison. *Radiographics* 2007; **27**: 237–57.

43. Miettinen M and Lasota J. Gastrointestinal stromal tumors: review on morphology, molecular pathology, prognosis, and differential diagnosis. *Arch Pathol Lab Med* 2006; **130**: 1466–78.

44. Perez EA, Livingstone AS, Franceschi D *et al.* Current incidence and outcomes of gastrointestinal mesenchymal tumors including gastrointestinal stromal tumors. *J Am Coll Surg* 2006; **202**: 623–9.

3

Endoscopy in the diagnosis and treatment of gastric cancer

Hiroyuki Osawa and Hironori Yamamoto

Introduction

Because of its lethal prognosis when advanced, early detection and resection of gastric cancer remains the best means of treating this neoplasm. In the hope of detecting this cancer in its earliest possible form, chromoendoscopy with indigo carmine spray was developed. This technique enhances fine surface structures and color contrast of the mucosa, resulting in improved diagnostic accuracy [1]. Since the late 1990s, advances in biomedical optics have been applied to overcome the limitations of chromoendoscopy for detecting various gastrointestinal (GI) diseases. Endoscopists require meticulous endoscopic technique and considerable clinical experience in diagnosing early gastric cancer (EGC). New and improved endoscopic modalities are being developed for screening high-risk patients.

The flexible spectral imaging color enhancement (FICE) system was introduced in 2005 as a novel image-processing tool for video endoscopy [2, 3, 4, 5]. FICE enhances the contrast of the gastric mucosal surface without the use of dyes. Because image processing can be executed using the endoscope processor, FICE does not require modification of the light source as does the narrow band imaging (NBI) system. Additionally, FICE provides optimal band images with the same light intensity as the conventional endoscope. Indeed, FICE can facilitate detection of changes in EGC without magnification and can accurately confirm the diagnosis of cancer with 40-fold magnification.

After an endoscopically detailed examination has been performed and the patient meets inclusion criteria, endoscopic therapy of EGC can be performed with the expectation of a complete cure [6]. Despite its lack of invasiveness, well-selected patients treated with endoscopic therapy should have outcomes comparable to those receiving operative therapy. Indeed, the 5-year survival rates for patients with EGC approaches 90%–100% in Japan [7, 8, 9, 10].

There are various types of endoscopic treatment available for gastric cancer, which can be classified as: tissue-destructive treatments, such as laser or argon plasma coagulation (APC) [11, 12], and endoscopic resection, such as endoscopic mucosal resection (EMR). When performed as a curative treatment, endoscopic resection is more advantageous than tissue-destructive treatments, because endoscopic resection allows the pathology of the affected tissue to be examined and hence the completeness of tumor resection can be assessed. Precise histopathological diagnosis of the resected specimen is important, because determining the depth of invasion and the presence or absence of lymphatic invasion indicates whether additional surgical treatment is necessary.

Endoscopic submucosal dissection (ESD) was developed in the early 2000s as a more reliable method of endoscopic resection than EMR [13, 14, 15]. In Japan, ESD has now been officially approved as an endoscopic treatment for EGC and the standard of care for EGC has shifted from EMR to ESD. Understanding the advantages of ESD compared with conventional EMR has led to its widespread use.

In this chapter, advances in endoscopic diagnosis of EGCs and their endoscopic therapies will be reviewed, highlighting developments in FICE and ESD.

Endoscopic diagnosis of early gastric cancer

General principles

Modest changes in the morphology and color of the mucosa are important factors for the diagnosis of EGC. The morphologic characteristics of EGC include mild elevation and shallow depression of the mucosa, as well as discontinuity with surrounding mucosa and areas of uneven surface. When the mucosa shows pale redness or fading of color, this indicates significant disease. Gastric cancer can be classified macroscopically according to the Japanese Classification of Gastric Carcinoma [16] or the Paris Endoscopic Classification of Superficial Neoplastic Lesions [17]. The Paris Classification resulted from a workshop that explored the utility and clinical relevance of the Japanese Classification. According to these classifications, gastric cancer can be categorized into six types, from type 0 to type 5. Early gastric cancers belong to the type 0 morphology and can be subclassified as indicated in Table 3.1 [18].

Table 3.1. Macroscopic types of gastric cancer

Type	Japanese classification	Paris classification
0	Superficial, flat tumors with or without minimal elevation or depression	Superficial polypoid, flat/depressed, or excavated tumors
0I	Protruded	Polypoid
0 IIa	Superficial and elevated	Non-polypoid and non-excavated, slightly elevated
0 IIb	Superficial and depressed	Non-polypoid and non-excavated, slightly depressed without ulcer
0 IIc	Superficial and depressed	Non-polypoid and non-excavated, slightly depressed without ulcer
0 III	Excavated	Non-polypoid with a frank ulcer
1	Polypoid tumors that are sharply demarcated from the surrounding mucosa and are usually attached on a wide base	Polypoid carcinomas that are usually attached on a wide base
2	Ulcerated carcinomas that have sharply demarcated and raised margins	Ulcerated carcinomas that have sharply demarcated and raised margins
3	Ulcerated carcinomas that have no definite limits and infiltrate into the surrounding wall	Ulcerated, infiltrating carcinomas that have no definite limits
4	Diffusely infiltrating carcinomas in which ulceration is not usually a marked feature	Non-ulcerated, diffusely infiltrating carcinomas
5	Carcinomas that cannot be classified into any of the above types	Unclassifiable advanced carcinomas

According to the Japanese Classification of Gastric Carcinoma [16], for the combined superficial types, the type occupying the largest area should be described first, followed by the next type (e.g., IIc+III). Types 0I and 0IIa are distinguished from each other by lesion thickness: type-0I lesions have a thickness more than twice that of the normal mucosa and type-0IIa lesions have a thickness up to twice that of the normal mucosa. Modified from data presented in the Japanese Classification of Gastric Carcinoma [16] and the Paris Endoscopic Classification of Superficial Neoplastic Lesions [17].

Flexible spectral imaging color enhancement (FICE) system as an endoscopic diagnostic tool

Instrumentation

Flexible spectral imaging color enhancement (FICE) is an endoscopic technique that was developed to enhance the capillary and the pit patterns of the gastric mucosa. FICE technology is based on the selection of spectral transmittance with a dedicated wavelength (Table 3.2). In contrast to NBI, in which the bandwidth of the spectral transmittance is narrowed by optical filters, FICE is based on a new spectral estimation technique that eliminates the need for optical filters. FICE takes an ordinary endoscopic image from a video processor and arithmetically processes the reflected photons to reconstitute virtual images at a choice of different wavelengths. Because the spectra of pixels are known, it is possible to depict the gastric mucosa on a single wavelength. These single-wavelength images are randomly selected, and assigned to red (R), green (G), and blue (B) to build and display a FICE-enhanced color image (Figure 3.1).

Instrument specifications and selection of optimal band images

Endoscopes used with the FICE system include EG-590ZW for routine and magnifying observation, EG-590WR for routine observation, and EG-530N for transnasal observation, all of which have been developed by Fujinon Corporation (Saitama, Japan) for the upper GI tract. They all require an electronic endoscope system (FTS4400 and 4500, Fujinon) (Figure 3.2). The EG-590ZW scope can magnify

Table 3.2. Initial setting patterns of wavelengths available in the FICE system

Set number	Blue	Green	Red
0	415	445	500
1	420	470	500
2	470	500	550
3	420	490	540
4	405	500	520
5	420	480	500
6	460	520	580
7	400	450	520
8	415	415	540
9	400	500	550

endoscopic images optically up to 135-fold [19, 20] through the use of a zoom attachment. It is easy to change wavelengths during each endoscopic procedure, because the system allows selection of a setting from up to ten possible wavelengths (Figure 3.3).

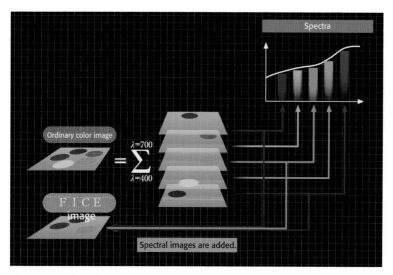

Figure 3.1. Principle of the newly developed flexible spectral imaging color enhancement (FICE) system to obtain the optimal band images. The spectral image for each wavelength is produced through the reflectance spectrum estimation technique from an ordinary endoscopy image obtained by white light illumination. Three spectral images are selected and allocated to RGB television signals to reconstruct the image.

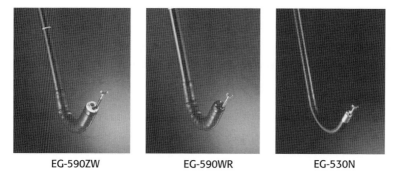

Figure 3.2. Endoscopes used with FICE system include EG-590ZW for routine and magnifying observation, EG-590WR for routine observation, and EG-530N for transnasal observation, all of which are developed by Fujinon Corporation for the upper gastrointestinal tract.

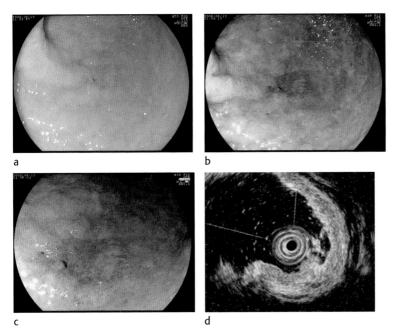

Figure 3.3a–d. **(a) Conventional endoscopic image of depressed-type cancer in the angulus. (b) Non-magnified FICE image of the same lesion. The cancer was reddish and surrounding normal mucosa was yellowish. (c) Forty-fold magnified FICE image showing cancer with finer pit pattern and linear-type irregular microvascular pattern (IMVP). The demarcation line between cancerous and non-cancerous mucosa was clearly identified. (d) Endoscopic ultrasonography (EUS) showed mucosal lesion without invasion to the submucosal layer.**

At the Jichi Medical University in Japan, Osawa *et al.*, as part of their endoscopic protocol for EGC detection, select the setting that best enhances the demarcation lines between cancerous lesions and surrounding areas without magnification [19, 20]. For most cases of gastric cancer, the best images are obtained utilizing the following three wavelengths: 470 nm for blue (B), 500 nm for green (G), and 550 nm for red (R). Other sets of wavelengths can also be easily selected during endoscopy in order to enhance vascular images or observe non-cancerous lesions.

FICE images of EGC without magnification

The characteristic finding of depressed-type EGC (Figure 3.4) on non-magnification views is a reddish lesion distinct from the surrounding yellowish normal mucosa. Conventional images are inferior to those generated by the FICE system because the latter technique optimizes visualization of the demarcation line between the cancer and surrounding mucosa. Conventional endoscopic images (Figure 3.4a)

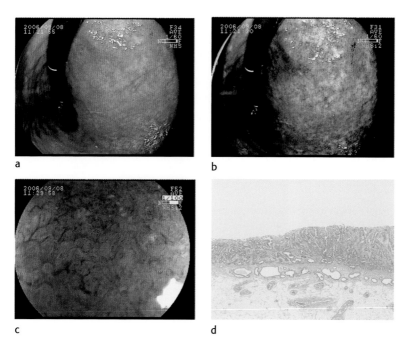

Figure 3.4a–d. (a) Conventional endoscopic images provide little information regarding depressed lesions located in the tangential line. (b) Non-magnified FICE image enhances the color contrast of such lesions, which enables easy diagnosis of EGC. (c) Forty-fold magnified FICE image showing cancer with linear-type IMVP. (d) Histological findings of the resected specimen. Well-differentiated adenocarcinoma with slightly depressed area was seen in the mucosa. (H&E, orig. mag. ×40).

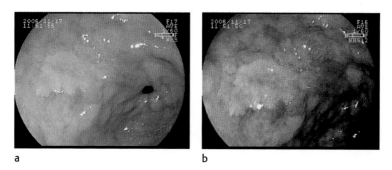

Figure 3.5a,b. (a) Some depressed cancers as shown in this case were recognized as whitish lesions by conventional endoscopy. (b) FICE images enhanced this lesion, leading to a clear demarcation line between the whitish cancerous lesion and the surrounding mucosa.

provide little information concerning depressed lesions viewed tangentially. FICE enhances the color contrast of these lesions, which facilitates the diagnosis of depressed-type EGC (Figure 3.4b). Some depressed cancers shown as whitish lesions on conventional endoscopy (Figure 3.5a) can be enhanced by FICE images (Figure 3.5b). FICE images can enhance the color contrast of these depressed lesions with other sets of wavelengths [420 nm (B), 490 nm (G), and 540 nm (R)] even using a small-caliber scope (EG-530N) (Figure 3.6).

Elevated-type EGCs on FICE images are depicted as yellowish lesions with a clearly contrasting demarcation line between the neoplastic lesion and the surrounding whitish atrophic mucosa (Figures 3.7 and 3.8). In some cases, a partially reddish patch is identified on the tumor surface similar to that more commonly seen in depressed-type EGC (Figure 3.9) [19].

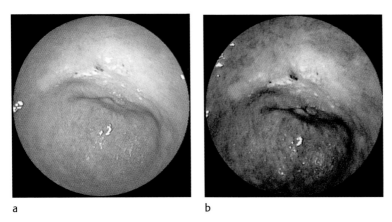

a   b

Figure 3.6a,b. (a) Conventional image with small-caliber-size scope (EG-530N) shows depressed-type cancer as a whitish lesion in the antrum. (b) FICE enhanced the color contrast of such a lesion with another set of wavelengths including 420 nm (B), 490 nm (G), and 540 nm (R) even using the small-caliber-size endoscope.

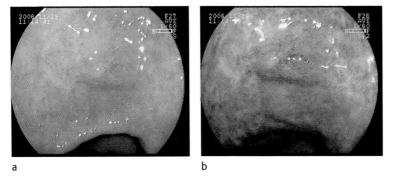

a   b

Figure 3.7a,b. (a) Conventional endoscopic image of elevated-type cancer in the body. (b) With FICE image, this cancer was detected easily as yellowish lesions with clearly contrasting demarcation lines between cancerous lesions and surrounding whitish atrophic mucosa.

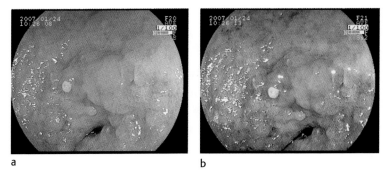

a   b

Figure 3.8a,b. (a) Conventional endoscopic image of elevated-type cancer in the antrum. (b) FICE provided more contrasting image between cancerous lesion and the surrounding atrophic mucosa. Cancerous lesion was shown as a finer pit pattern (Table 3.3).

Table 3.3. FICE images of gastric cancer with half magnification

Irregular microstructural pattern of tumor surface

1. Non-structure pattern
2. Finer structure pattern
3. Large and small pit pattern
4. Tubular pit pattern
5. Multiple structure pattern

Irregular microvascular pattern of tumor surface

1. Small dot pattern
2. Linear pattern
3. Twig pattern

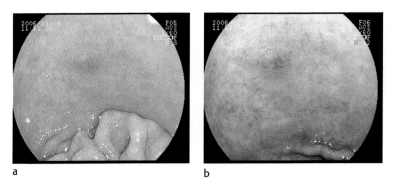

a   b

Figure 3.9a,b. (a) Conventional endoscopic image of elevated-type cancer in the antrum. (b) FICE image enhanced a reddish area on the tumor surface, similar to a depressed-type cancer.

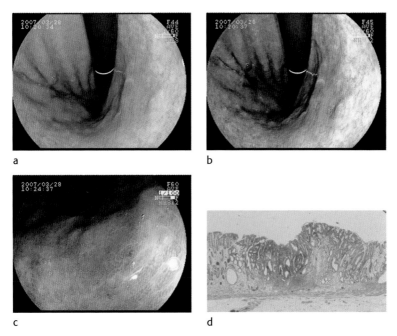

a   b

c   d

Figure 3.10a–d. **The FICE system is quite useful for the detection of minute gastric cancer.**
(a) Conventional endoscopic image of elevated-type minute cancer in the body. (b) FICE image
enhanced a reddish area on the tumor surface. (c) A 30-fold magnified FICE image showed
irregular microstructural pattern with large and small pits, suggesting a cancer. (d) Histological
findings of the resected specimen. Well-differentiated adenocarcinoma 4 mm in diameter was seen
in the mucosa. (H&E, orig. mag. ×40.) The size of the pathologic lesion was consistent with that of
the FICE image.

The FICE system is quite useful for the detection of minute (≤5 mm) gastric cancers, even without magnification (Figure 3.10). The new contrast-enhanced images obtained with the FICE system have the potential to increase the detection rate of gastric cancers and provide more effective screening.

FICE images of EGC with magnification

Magnification of FICE (Figure 3.11) images is quite useful for the accurate diagnosis of EGC [19]. The irregular microstructural or non-structural patterns as well as the irregular microvascular patterns seen in all morphologic types of EGC are clearly identified on the tumor surface with 40-fold magnification (Figure 3.12; see also Figures 3.4, 3.5, 3.11). The intramucosal vascular pattern is closely related to the depth of vertical cancer invasion. Large irregular vessels on the tumor surface are observed in many cases of EGC with submucosal invasion (see Figure 3.11c and d). These observations are helpful in confirming the endoscopic diagnosis of EGC.

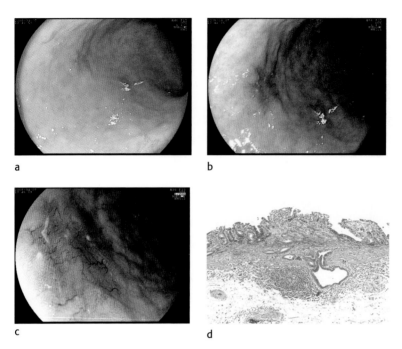

a   b

c   d

Figure 3.11a–d. The presence and pattern of IMVP are closely related to the depth of vertical cancer invasion. Large irregular vessels on the tumor surface, especially twig patterns, are observed in many cases of EGC with pathologically submucosal invasion. (a) Conventional endoscopic image of depressed-type cancer in the body. (b) FICE showed more contrasting image between the cancerous lesion and the surrounding mucosa than conventional scope. (c) A 30-fold magnified FICE image showed the twig pattern of IMVP, suggesting an invasion to the submucosal layer. (d) Histological findings of the resected specimen. Well-differentiated adenocarcinoma was seen in the mucosa and invaded to the partially submucosal layer, consistent with the twig pattern of the FICE image.

Determination of the extent of EGC

Even though targeted areas of the mucosa can be removed with precision with ESD, a complete resection cannot be assured without determining the full lateral extent of EGCs. The margin of the tumor should be carefully determined because the actual tumor margin may be wider than suspected on conventional endoscopy. Chromoendoscopy is performed by spraying dyes such as indigo carmine on the mucosa after thoroughly washing the mucus. This technique is useful in determining the lateral tumor extent.

Tumor margins are easily identified on FICE images even without magnification, as EGCs are highlighted by surrounding whitish atrophic mucosa. Also, magnified

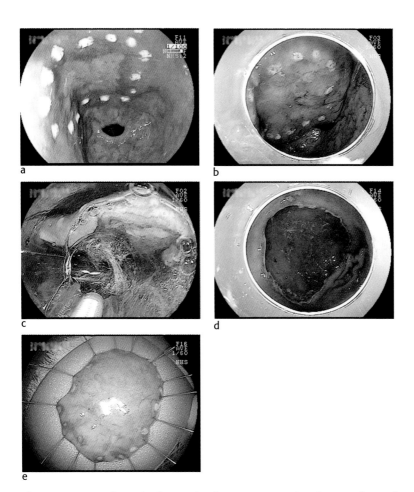

Figure 3.12a–e. Endoscopic pictures showing an ESD procedure for an early gastric cancer at the antrum. Resected specimen showing a complete en-bloc resection of the entire lesion. (a) Several marks are placed at the surrounding intact mucosa on the circumference about 5 mm outside the tumor margin. The tumor margin was clearly identified with the FICE image. (b) The tumor and the surrounding incision line are elevated by submucosal injection of sodium hyaluronate solution. (c) Submucosal dissection with a needle knife. Submucosal tissue with a blood vessel is clearly visualized by opening the mucosal incision with the tip of the ST hood. (d) Mucosal defect after ESD. ESD was completed without complications.

images with FICE or NBI can depict the fine mucosal and vascular changes that accompany EGC [19, 20, 21, 22]. With the FICE system and 40-fold magnification, irregular microstructural or non-structural patterns are also routinely found within cancerous lesions but not the surrounding mucosa [19, 20]. This technique may clearly show the margin between tumor and uninvolved mucosa even when this margin is blurred on conventional images. Low-magnification settings on the FICE system allow endoscopists to more easily maintain the proper distance between the tip of the endoscope and the gastric mucosa. Low magnification also permits inspection of broad areas of the gastric mucosa that include both cancerous and surrounding non-cancerous portions on the same endoscopic images. These findings are also helpful in accurately confirming the demarcation line of the tumor, assisting ESD so that en-bloc specimens with free lateral margins can be achieved (Figure 3.12).

Determination of the depth of tumor invasion

Tumor depth staging of EGC on conventional endoscopy has an accuracy of between 70% and 80%. Mucosal cancers include: small protruded type (type 0I); superficial elevated type (type 0IIa) with smooth surface; and small shallow depressed type (type 0IIc). Submucosal invasion is suspected if either an irregularly shaped nodule on the margin or interrupted large folds are discovered. Advanced gastric cancer (AGC) involves ulcerative lesions with a surrounding tumor mound or those with folds that are elevated and merged [23, 24].

The depth of invasion of EGCs strongly correlates with lymph node metastasis so that pretreatment depth staging is important. Conventional endoscopy and endoscopic ultrasonography (EUS) have proven useful for tumor staging (see Chapter 7) [23, 24, 25, 26, 27]. FICE with magnification shows the large irregular vessels on the tumor surface that typically accompany submucosal invasion (see Figure 3.11).

Endoscopic ultrasonography is most useful for determining the depth of invasion in small elevated-type differentiated cancer [26]. Endosonographic irregular narrowing and a budding sign of more than 1 mm in depth in the third layer (submucosa) should raise suspicion of submucosal invasion in EGC even in the absence of ulceration on conventional endoscopy [27]. EUS is also useful for evaluating perigastric lymph node metastasis and direct infiltration to the adjacent organs (see Chapter 7) [25].

Endoscopic therapy for early gastric cancer

General principles

Endoscopic therapy for EGC has the great advantage of avoiding both a laparoscopic and an open surgical procedure. When selecting patients for endoscopic therapy, it is important that the efficacy of tumor extirpation and outcomes are comparable to those of more invasive procedures. Thus, very strict selection criteria are mandatory before endoscopic therapy is chosen. Detailed pathologic examination of the resected tissue is required to ensure that the cancer has been completely resected. Additional therapy may be needed if the specimen margins are not tumor free. The most important factor influencing the survival of patients with EGC is the presence or absence of lymph node metastasis [9, 10, 28, 29]. The incidence of lymph node metastasis has been reported as 1%–3% for mucosal cancers and 11%–20% for submucosal cancers in the stomach [28]. Therefore, endoscopic therapy should only be used for EGCs when the risk of lymph node metastasis is negligible and a cure is expected after complete local resection.

Gastric cancer treatment guidelines

Endoscopic submucosal dissection has recently been established as a more reliable tissue-retrieving endoscopic therapy than EMR. ESD allows endoscopists to incise and remove the affected mucosa using a variety of endoscopic electrosurgical knives. Unlike snaring, which is the mainstay of EMR [30], ESD enables en-bloc resection of the affected mucosa in a more reliable manner, regardless of the size of the affected mucosa [31, 32, 33, 34, 35]. It is important to note, however, that even though ESD permits local en-bloc resection of larger EGCs, criteria other than tumor size (i.e., infiltration depth, ulceration, and tumor differentiation) must still be considered. Therefore, patients who have lesions with a high risk for lymph node metastasis are still not candidates for endoscopic therapy, even though local en-bloc resection is technically possible.

The effectiveness of ESD must be judged by histologic evaluation of the resected specimen. Additional gastrectomy with lymph node dissection is required if submucosal invasion or vessel permeation can be identified in the endoscopically resected specimen [36, 37, 38].

The range of extended indications currently considered in Japan

Based on the reports by Gotoda *et al.* at the National Cancer Center and other groups [39], current indications for ESD in Japan include: (1) non-ulcerated, differentiated-type mucosal carcinomas regardless of tumor size; and (2) differentiated-type mucosal carcinomas with an ulcer scar ≤ 30 mm. Lesions that meet the above criteria should be resected endoscopically in one piece. Resected tissues are sectioned at 2-mm intervals for pathologic evaluation. ESD or EMR can be regarded as curative when a differentiated-type mucosal carcinoma without submucosal invasion or lymphatic or venous invasion is completely resected with a tumor-free margin.

According to the report from the National Cancer Center, no lymph node metastases were found in 1230 intramucosal cancers ≤ 3 cm in size without lymphatic or venous invasion, regardless of the presence of ulceration. Irrespective of tumor size, 929 differentiated adenocarcinomas without ulceration, lymphatic or venous invasion did not show lymph node involvement.

Endoscopic submucosal dissection

Endoscopic submucosal dissection is a novel technique that allows for larger, more definitive resections than conventional EMR, thereby expanding the indications for endoscopic treatment of EGCs. Hirao *et al.* were the first to report incising the surrounding mucosa of the lesion using a needle knife for precise determination of the area to be removed [40]. ESD involves a mucosal incision around the lesion and subsequent submucosal dissection for the removal of mucosa using electrosurgical knives. Once the tumor margin has been marked by magnifying endoscopy and/or chromoendoscopy, the mucosa can be incised, resulting in a high probability of resecting lesions in one piece regardless of tumor size or location (Figure 3.12). ESD, however, requires more endoscopic skill and takes longer to perform than snaring employed with EMR [30, 31, 32, 33, 34, 35, 41, 42].

The first step in ESD is to place several marks with the tip of the knife using coagulation current on the surrounding intact mucosa leaving a tumor-free margin of at least 5 mm. Then both the cancer and tumor-free margin are elevated by submucosal injection of physiological saline or sodium hyaluronate solution. Sodium hyaluronate solution can maintain submucosal elevation for a longer time and is preferable for providing safe margins with the muscularis propria for the incision and dissection of the mucosa [32, 33, 43, 44, 45]. Small amounts of epinephrine and indigo carmine are often mixed into the local injection fluid.

Various endoscopic dissection instruments such as a needle knife allow mucosal incision along the outside of the marks, insertion of a knife through the incised layer of mucosa, and subsequent dissection of the submucosal tissue. This method enables the removal of the mucosal lesion in one piece by dissecting the entire submucosal layer. Several knives and hoods are available for ESD in Japan at the present time. The major tools for ESD are shown in Figure 3.13.

(a) Needle knife (KD-10Q-1; Olympus, Tokyo, Japan)
(b) IT knife (KD-610L; Olympus, Tokyo, Japan) [31, 41, 42]
(c) Hook knife (KD-620LR; Olympus, Tokyo, Japan) [34]
(d) Flex knife (KD-630L; Olympus, Tokyo, Japan) [35]
(e) Triangle-tip knife (KD-640L; Olympus, Tokyo, Japan)

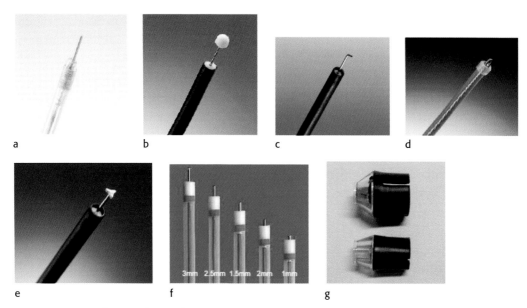

a   b   c   d

e   f   g

Figure 3.13a–g. Endoscopic devices for ESD. (a) Needle knife (KD-10Q-1; Olympus, Tokyo, Japan).
(b) IT knife (KD-610L; Olympus, Tokyo, Japan) [31, 41, 42]. (c) Hook knife (KD-620LR; Olympus, Tokyo,
Japan) [34]. (d) Flex knife (KD-630L; Olympus, Tokyo, Japan) [35]. (e) Triangle-tip knife (KD-640L;
Olympus, Tokyo, Japan). (f) Flush knife (DK2618JN; Fujifilm, Tokyo, Japan). (g) ST hood (DH-15GR;
Fujifilm, Tokyo, Japan) [32].

(f) Flush knife (DK2618JN; Fujifilm, Tokyo, Japan)

(g) ST hood (DH-15GR; Fujifilm, Tokyo, Japan) [32]

Handling of resected specimens

According to the Second English Edition of the Japanese Classification of Gastric
Carcinoma [16], specimens obtained by endoscopic or laparoscopic mucosal resection should be handled in the following manner: the specimen should be spread
out, pinned on a flat cork, and fixed in formalin solution. The size of specimen, the
size and shape of the tumor, and the margins should be recorded on a schematic
diagram. The proximal cut end is indicated by an arrow, if possible. Fixed materials
should be sectioned serially at 2-mm intervals parallel to a line that includes the
closest resection margin of the specimen.

Histologic examination

The histologic type and the size of the largest dimension of the tumor, the presence or absence of ulceration (UL), lymphatic invasion (ly), and venous invasion

(v) should be recorded. The depth of invasion (M, SM1, SM2) is determined and recorded only when the vertical margin (VM) is negative (SM1, submucosal invasion < 0.5 mm; SM2, invasion ≥ 0.5 mm).

The lateral margin (LM) should be assessed, and, if negative, the length (mm) of the free margin or the number of normal tubules in the margin is recorded. Tumor extent, together with depth of invasion, should be recorded on a schematic diagram.

The resection is regarded as curative if the following criteria are met: depth M (confined to mucosa), histologically papillary adenocarcinoma (pap) or tubular adenocarcinoma (tub), no ulcer or ulcer scar in the tumor, negative VM, no tumor cells within 1 mm of LM, and no lymphatic or venous invasion.

There are differences between Japanese and Western classification systems used to define the pathology of early forms of GI cancers [46, 47, 48]. These differences have made it difficult for Western endoscopists to extrapolate to their own practices the outcomes of EMR reported in Japanese studies. Efforts are ongoing among pathologists to correlate the two classifications [17, 49].

Summary

Early detection is essential for improving outcomes in patients with gastric cancer. With earlier detection, the likelihood of cure with non-surgical endoscopic therapy increases. The FICE system provides better information on the tumor margin as well as abnormal surface structures in EGC. Accordingly, it is probably the best single examination for EGC detection. When choosing a therapeutic approach, the absolute depth of mural penetration by the tumor and the presence or absence of nodal involvement are vital for assigning patients to surgical or non-surgical endoscopic therapy.

When considering endoscopic resection, histologic type is also an important consideration, as patients with differentiated-type mucosal carcinoma are better suited to endoscopic therapy. In properly selected patients, endoscopic therapy of EGC can provide a cure rate equivalent to that of surgical resection. It is imperative to select the appropriate technique to achieve the highest possible cure rate.

Endoscopic submucosal dissection has been developed as a reliable technique for en-bloc resection, and its therapeutic effectiveness is increasing. It is important to resect the tumor completely in one piece and to confirm that the tumor is a differentiated-type mucosal carcinoma without lymphatic or venous invasion. If a complete cure is not obtained, additional surgical therapy should be considered.

REFERENCES

1. Triantafillidis JK and Cheracakis P. Diagnostic evaluation of patients with EGC – a literature review. *Hepatogastroenterology* 2004; **51**: 618–24.

2. Miyake Y, Sekiya T, Kubo S *et al.* A new spectrophotometer for measuring the spectral reflectance of gastric mucous membrane. *J Photogr Sci* 1989; **37**: 134–8.

3. Shiobara T, Zhou H, Haneishi N *et al.* Improved color reproduction of electronic endoscopes. *J Imaging Sci Technol* 1996; **40**: 494–501.

4. Tsumura N, Tanaka T, Haneishi H *et al.* Optimal design of mosaic color electronic endoscopes. *Opt Commun* 1998; **145**: 27–32.

5. Shiobara T, Haneishi N, and Miyake Y. Color correction for colorimetric color reproduction in an electronic endoscope. *Opt Commun* 1995; **114**: 57–63.

6. Nishi M, Omori Y, and Miwa K (eds.). *Japanese Classification of Gastric Carcinoma*, 1st edn. Tokyo: Kanehara & Co. Ltd./Japanese Research Society for Gastric Cancer, 1995.

7. Onodera H, Tokunaga A, Yoshiyuki T *et al.* Surgical outcome of 483 patients with EGC: prognosis, postoperative morbidity and mortality, and gastric remnant cancer. *Hepatogastroenterology* 2004; **51**: 82–5.

8. Inoue K, Tobe T, Kan N *et al.* Problems in the definition and treatment of EGC. *Br J Surg* 1991; **78**: 818–21.

9. Maehara Y, Orita H, Okuyama T *et al.* Predictors of lymph node metastasis in EGC. *Br J Surg* 1992; **79**: 245–7.

10. Seto Y, Nagawa H and Muto T. Impact of lymph node metastasis on survival with EGC. *World J Surg* 1997; **21**: 186–9.

11. Sagawa T, Takayama T, Oku T *et al.* Argon plasma coagulation for successful treatment of EGC with intramucosal invasion. *Gut* 2003; **52**: 334–9.

12. Murakami M, Nishino K, Inoue A *et al.* Argon plasma coagulation for the treatment of EGC. *Hepatogastroenterology* 2004; **51**: 1658–61.

13. Gotoda T, Yamamoto H, and Soetikno RM. Endoscopic submucosal dissection of early gastric cancer. *J Gastroenterol* 2006; **41**: 929–42.

14. Yamamoto H. Mucosectomy in the colon with endoscopic submucosal dissection. *Endoscopy* 2005; **37**: 764–8.

15. Yamamoto H. Endoscopic submucosal dissection of early cancers and large flat adenomas. *Clin Gastroenterol Hepatol* 2005; **3** Suppl 1: S67–70.

16. Japanese Gastric Cancer Association. Japanese Classification of Gastric Carcinoma, second English edition. *Gastric Cancer* 1998; **1**: 10–24.

17. The Paris Endoscopic Classification of Superficial Neoplastic Lesions: esophagus, stomach, and colon: November 30 to December 1, 2002. *Gastrointest Endosc* 2003; **58** Suppl 6: S3–43.

18. Yamamoto H. Technology insight: endoscopic submucosal dissection of gastrointestinal neoplasms. *Nat Clin Pract Gastroenterol Hepatol* 2007; **4**: 511–20.

19. Osawa H, Yoshizawa M, Yamamoto H *et al.* Optimal band imaging system can facilitate detection of change in depressed type EGC. *Gastrointest Endosc* 2008; **67**: 226–34.

20. Yoshizawa M, Osawa H, Yamamoto H *et al.* Newly developed optimal band imaging system for the diagnosis of early gastric cancer. *Dig Endosc* 2008; **20**(4): 194–7.

21. Yao K, Oishi T, Matsui T *et al.* Novel magnified endoscopic findings of microvascular architecture in intramucosal gastric cancer. *Gastrointest Endosc* 2002; **56**: 279–84.

22. Sumiyama K, Kaise M, Nakayoshi T *et al.* Combined use of a magnifying endoscope with a narrow band imaging system and a multibending endoscope for en bloc EMR of early stage gastric cancer. *Gastrointest Endosc* 2004; **60**: 79–84.

23. Sano T, Okuyama Y, Kobori O *et al.* EGC: endoscopic diagnosis of depth of invasion. *Dig Dis Sci* 1990; **35**: 1340–4.

24. Yanai H, Matsumoto Y, Harada T *et al.* Endoscopic ultrasonography and endoscopy for staging depth of invasion in EGC: a pilot study. *Gastrointest Endosc* 1997; **46**: 212–16.

25. Akahoshi K, Misawa T, Fujishima H *et al.* Preoperative evaluation of gastric cancer by endoscopic ultrasound. *Gut* 1991; **32**: 479–82.

26. Akahoshi K, Chijiwa Y, Hamada S *et al.* Pretreatment staging of endoscopically early gastric cancer with a 15 MHz ultrasound catheter probe. *Gastrointest Endosc* 1998; **48**: 470–6.

27. Matsumoto Y, Yanai H, Tokiyama H *et al.* Endoscopic ultrasonography for diagnosis of submucosal invasion in EGC. *J Gastroenterol* 2000; **35**: 326–31.

28. Adachi Y, Shiraishi N and Kitano S. Modern treatment of EGC: review of the Japanese experience. *Dig Surg* 2002; **19**: 333–9.

29. Kunisaki C, Shimada H, Takahashi M *et al.* Prognostic factors in EGC. *Hepatogastroenterology* 2001; **48**: 294–8.

30. Kumai K. Indications of endoscopic submucosal dissection for early gastroenterological cancer: advantages and disadvantages (in Japanese with English abstract). *Endosc Dig* 2004; **16**: 703–8.

31. Ono H, Kondo H, Gotoda T *et al.* Endoscopic mucosal resection for treatment of EGC. *Gut* 2001; **48**: 225–9.

32. Yamamoto H, Kawata H, Sunada K *et al.* Successful en-bloc resection of large superficial tumours in the stomach and colon using sodium hyaluronate and small-calibre-tip transparent hood. *Endoscopy* 2003; **35**: 690–4.

33. Yamamoto H, Sekine Y, Higashizawa T *et al.* Successful en bloc resection of a large superficial gastric cancer by using sodium hyaluronate and electrocautery incision forceps. *Gastrointest Endosc* 2001; **54**: 629–32.

34. Oyama T and Kikuchi Y. Aggressive endoscopic mucosal resection in the upper GI tract – Hook knife method. *Minim Invasive Ther Allied Technol* 2002; **11**: 291–5.

35. Yahagi N, Fujishiro M, Imagawa A *et al.* Endoscopic submucosal dissection for the reliable en bloc resection of colorectal mucosal tumours. *Dig Endosc* 2004; **16**: S89–S92.

36. Rembacken BJ, Gotoda T, Fujii T and Axon AT. Endoscopic mucosal resection. *Endoscopy* 2001; **33**: 709–18.

37. Borie F, Rigau V, Fingerhut A and Millat B. French Association for Surgical Research. Prognostic factors for EGC in France: Cox regression analysis of 332 cases. *World J Surg* 2004; **28**: 686–91.

38. Pelz J, Merkel S, Horbach T *et al.* Determination of nodal status and treatment in EGC. *Eur J Surg Oncol* 2004; **30**: 935–41.

39. Gotoda T, Yanagisawa A, Sasako M *et al.* Incidence of lymph node metastasis from EGC: estimation with a large number of cases at two large centers. *Gastric Cancer* 2000; **3**: 219–25.

40. Hirao M, Masuda K, Asanuma T *et al.* Endoscopic resection of early gastric cancer and other tumors with local injection of hypertonic saline-epinephrine. *Gastrointest Endosc* 1988; **34**: 264–9.

41. Ohkuwa M, Hosokawa K, Boku N *et al.* New endoscopic treatment for intramucosal gastric tumours using an insulated-tip diathermic knife. *Endoscopy* 2001; **33**: 221–6.

42. Rosch T, Sarbia M, Schumacher B *et al.* Attempted endoscopic en bloc resection of mucosal and submucosal tumours using insulated-tip knives: a pilot series. *Endoscopy* 2004; **36**: 788–801.

43. Fujishiro M, Yahagi N, Kashimura K *et al.* Different mixtures of sodium hyaluronate and their ability to create submucosal fluid cushions for endoscopic mucosal resection. *Endoscopy* 2004; **36**: 584–9.

44. Yamamoto H, Yube T, Isoda N *et al.* A novel method of endoscopic mucosal resection using sodium hyaluronate. *Gastrointest Endosc* 1999; **50**: 251–6.

45. Fujishiro M, Yahagi N, Kashimura K *et al.* Comparison of various submucosal injection solutions for maintaining mucosal elevation during endoscopic mucosal resection. *Endoscopy* 2004; **36**: 579–83.

46. Schlemper RJ, Itabashi M, Kato Y *et al.* Differences in diagnostic criteria for gastric carcinoma between Japanese and western pathologists. *Lancet* 1997; **349**: 1725–9 (erratum in *Lancet* 1997; **350**: 524).

47. Schlemper RJ, Itabashi M, Kato Y *et al.* Differences in the diagnostic criteria used by Japanese and Western pathologists to diagnose colorectal carcinoma. *Cancer* 1998; **82**: 60–9.

48. Schlemper RJ, Dawsey SM, Itabashi M *et al.* Differences in diagnostic criteria for esophageal squamous cell carcinoma between Japanese and Western pathologists. *Cancer* 2000; **88**: 996–1006.

49. Schlemper RJ, Riddell RH, Kato Y *et al.* The Vienna classification of gastrointestinal epithelial neoplasia. *Gut* 2000; **47**: 251–5.

4

Upper gastrointestinal series in the diagnosis of gastric cancer

Marc S. Levine

Introduction

Although the incidence of gastric carcinoma has declined since the 1960s [1, 2], it continucs to be a deadly disease, with overall 5-year survival rates of less than 20% [3, 4]. There also has been a gradual shift in the distribution of gastric cancer from the antrum proximally to the fundus and cardia during this same period [5, 6]. As many as 40% of all gastric cancers are now located in the fundus or cardiac region [3, 4, 6]. This changing pattern of disease has major implications for the radio-logic diagnosis of gastric cancer, as the gastric cardia and fundus must be carefully evaluated in all patients with suspected gastric tumors. The double-contrast bar-ium study is a valuable technique for detection of tumors in the fundus that are inaccessible to manual palpation as well as scirrhous tumors encasing the wall of the stomach. Double-contrast studies are also particularly useful for the detection of early cancers, which have a much better prognosis than advanced cancers. This chapter reviews the role of barium studies in the diagnosis of gastric cancer.

Early gastric cancer

Early gastric cancers are defined histologically as tumors limited to the mucosa or submucosa, regardless of the presence or absence of regional lymph node metas-tases (which does not substantially affect the prognosis). Unlike advanced carcin-omas, which have a dismal prognosis, early gastric cancers are curable lesions, with 5-year survival rates of 90%–95% [7, 8, 9].

The double-contrast barium study has been widely recognized as a useful radio-logic technique for the diagnosis of early gastric cancer. The Japanese have been particularly successful in detecting early gastric cancer, using a combination of double-contrast barium studies and endoscopy. While early cancers are often detected in Japan, they are rarely diagnosed in the United States or other Western countries. This discrepancy can be attributed to mass screening of the adult population in Japan because of the high prevalence of gastric carcinoma in that country [7, 8]. Such screening studies are rarely performed in the West, however, because of the lower incidence of gastric cancer. Unfortunately, most patients with symptoms of gastric cancer have advanced tumors, so radiologists in the West are unlikely to detect early gastric cancers as long as these studies are performed predominantly on symptomatic patients [10].

Radiographic findings

The Japanese Endoscopic Society has divided early gastric cancers into three types (see Chapters 3 and 7) [11]. Type I cancers are elevated lesions that protrude more than 5 mm into the lumen. Type II cancers are superficial lesions that are further subdivided into three groups – types IIa, IIb, and IIc – depending on the morphologic features of the tumor. Type IIa lesions are elevated but protrude less than 5 mm into the lumen. Type IIb lesions are relatively flat. Type IIc lesions are slightly depressed but do not penetrate beyond the muscularis mucosae. Finally, type III lesions are true mucosal ulcers, with the ulcer penetrating beyond the muscularis mucosae into the submucosa but not the muscularis propria. When early gastric cancers exhibit more than one of these morphologic features, they may have a dual classification, with the predominant feature listed first (e.g., type I + IIc).

Type I early gastric cancers typically appear on double-contrast studies as small protruded lesions in the stomach [10, 12, 13] (Figure 4.1). Because adenomatous polyps can undergo malignant degeneration, the possibility of early gastric cancer should be suspected for any sessile or pedunculated polyps greater than 1 cm in size. Other relatively large polypoid masses that protrude considerably into the lumen can still be classified histologically as early cancers [13]. Thus, polypoid carcinomas cannot be diagnosed definitively as early or advanced lesions on the basis of the findings of barium studies.

Type II early gastric cancers are relatively flat lesions with elevated, superficial, or protruded components. These lesions may be manifested on double-contrast studies by plaque-like elevations, mucosal nodularity, shallow ulcers, or some combination of these findings (Figure 4.2) [10, 12, 13, 14]. Occasionally, these lesions can be quite extensive, involving a considerable surface area of the stomach without invading beyond the submucosa.

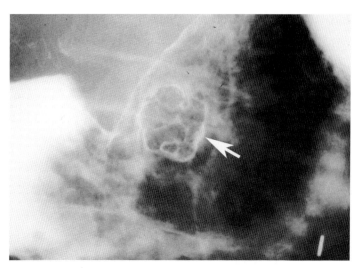

Figure 4.1. Early gastric cancer. A type I lesion is seen as a small polypoid mass (arrow) in the proximal gastric antrum near the lesser curvature.

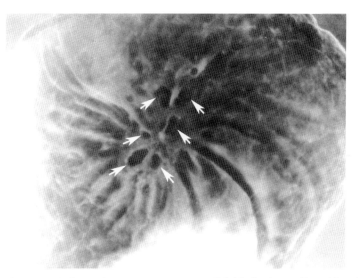

Figure 4.2. Early gastric cancer. A type II superficial lesion is manifested by a focal cluster of slightly elevated, irregular nodules (arrows) with folds radiating toward this central area of mucosal nodularity. Reproduced with permission [19].

Type III early gastric cancers usually appear on double-contrast studies as shallow ulcer craters with nodularity of the adjacent mucosa and clubbing or fusion of radiating folds due to infiltration of the adjoining folds by tumor (Figure 4.3) [12, 13]. Careful analysis of the findings usually permits differentiation from benign

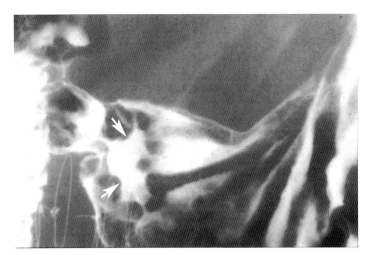

Figure 4.3. Early gastric cancer. A type III lesion is seen as a scalloped ulcer (arrows) in the distal gastric antrum with nodular, clubbed folds abutting the ulcer due to infiltration of the adjoining folds by tumor. Reproduced with permission [21].

gastric ulcers, which have different radiographic features (see below). Although some lesions with a suspicious appearance are found to be benign, endoscopy and biopsy are required for all lesions with equivocal radiographic findings in order to avoid missing early gastric cancers.

Advanced gastric cancer

Clinical findings

Most patients with gastric carcinoma become symptomatic only after they have advanced lesions with local or distant metastases. Common presenting findings include epigastric pain, bloating, or a palpable epigastric mass [15]. Other patients may have nausea and vomiting due to gastric outlet obstruction, early satiety due to linitis plastica, dysphagia due to cardia involvement, or signs and symptoms of upper gastrointestinal bleeding due to ulceration of the tumor. Still other patients with advanced gastric cancer may present with clinical signs of metastatic disease, such as anorexia, weight loss, jaundice, ascites, and hepatic enlargement.

Radiographic findings

Advanced gastric carcinomas can sometimes be recognized on abdominal radiographs by abnormalities of the gastric bubble in the left upper quadrant. Large polypoid lesions may produce a soft-tissue mass that indents the gastric shadow, whereas scirrhous carcinomas may produce a narrowed, tubular gas shadow, suggesting the diagnosis of linitis plastica. Rarely, mucin-producing scirrhous carcinomas may contain areas of calcification that have a stippled, punctate appearance [16]. When gastric carcinoma is suspected on the basis of abdominal radiographs, a barium study should be performed for a more certain diagnosis.

Concern about missing gastric cancer on barium studies has often been used as a rationale for performing endoscopy as the initial diagnostic test in patients with upper gastrointestinal symptoms. In one study, however, double-contrast examinations showed the lesion in 99% of patients with gastric carcinoma, and malignant tumor was diagnosed or suspected on the basis of the radiographic findings in 96% [17]. In the same study, endoscopy had been recommended to rule out malignant tumor in less than 5% of all patients who underwent double-contrast examinations. Thus, a high sensitivity can be achieved in the radiographic diagnosis of gastric carcinoma without exposing an inordinate number of patients to unnecessary endoscopy.

Advanced gastric carcinomas usually appear on barium studies as polypoid, ulcerative, or infiltrative lesions. However, many tumors have mixed morphologic features, so considerable overlap exists in the radiographic classification of these lesions. Scirrhous carcinomas and cardia carcinomas produce distinctive radiographic findings; these tumors are therefore discussed separately in later sections.

Polypoid carcinomas

Polypoid carcinomas usually appear radiographically as lobulated or fungating masses. On double-contrast studies, polypoid lesions on the dependent or posterior wall appear as filling defects in the barium pool, whereas polypoid lesions on the nondependent or anterior wall are etched in white by a thin layer of barium trapped between the edge of the mass and the adjacent mucosa (Figure 4.4). These lesions often contain irregular areas of ulceration due to necrosis of tumor. Bulky polypoid tumors may protrude substantially into the lumen but rarely cause gastric outlet obstruction. Occasionally, polypoid carcinomas of the antrum may prolapse through the pylorus into the duodenal bulb, appearing as mass lesions at the base of the bulb (Figure 4.5).

Ulcerated carcinomas

Ulcerated carcinomas are those in which the bulk of the tumor mass has been replaced by ulceration. These lesions are often called "malignant ulcers," but the

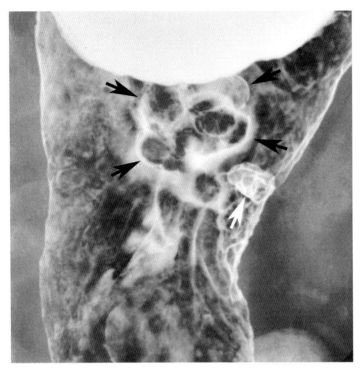

Figure 4.4. Polypoid gastric carcinoma. This patient has a polypoid mass on the posterior wall of the upper gastric body, manifested by multilobulated filling defects (black arrows) in the barium pool. A separate portion of the lesion is etched in white (white arrow) on the greater curvature.

term is a misnomer, as it is not the ulcer but the surrounding tumor that is malignant. Malignant ulcers classically appear en face as irregular ulcer craters eccentrically located within a rind of malignant tissue [18, 19]. There may be distortion or even obliteration of surrounding areae gastricae due to infiltration of the adjacent mucosa by tumor. Malignant ulcers often have scalloped, irregular borders, with thickened, lobulated, or clubbed folds abutting the ulcer due to infiltration of the adjoining folds by tumor (see Figure 4.3) [18, 19]. When viewed in profile, malignant ulcers are located within the expected contour of the stomach within a discrete tumor mass that forms acute angles with the adjacent gastric wall rather than the obtuse, gently sloping angles expected for a benign mound of edema (Figure 4.6) [18, 19].

In contrast, benign gastric ulcers viewed en face classically appear as round or ovoid ulcer niches, often associated with a smooth, surrounding mound of edema and/or regular, symmetric folds that radiate directly to the edge of the ulcer crater (Figure 4.7) [19, 20, 21]. When viewed in profile, benign ulcers project outside the

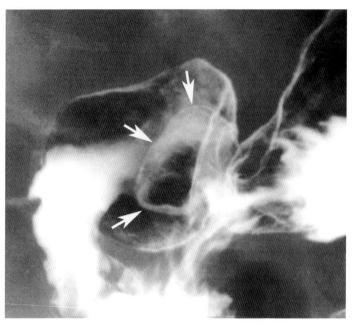

Figure 4.5. Prolapsed antral carcinoma. A smooth polypoid mass (arrows) is seen at the base of the duodenal bulb. Note how the mass is contiguous with the pylorus. This patient had an antral carcinoma that prolapsed into the duodenum.

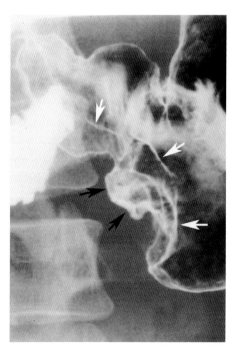

Figure 4.6. Malignant gastric ulcer. This patient has an ulcerated mass on the greater curvature of the gastric antrum. Note how the ulcer (black arrows) projects inside the lumen within a discrete mass that is etched in white (white arrows) and forms acute angles with the adjacent gastric wall. These findings are characteristic of a malignant ulcer viewed in profile.

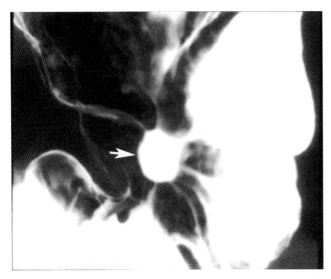

Figure 4.7. Benign gastric ulcer. An ovoid ulcer (arrow) is seen on the posterior wall of the gastric body with smooth, straight folds radiating directly to the edge of the ulcer crater. These findings are characteristic of a benign ulcer viewed en face.

contour of the adjacent gastric wall and are sometimes associated with a Hampton's line or an ulcer mound or collar (see Figure 4.8) [19, 20, 21].

Finally, equivocal ulcers are those that have mixed features of benign and malignant disease, so a confident diagnosis cannot be made on radiographic criteria. Features that place ulcers in this category include irregularity of ulcer shape, asymmetry of mass effect surrounding the ulcer, focal enlargement of surrounding areae gastricae (Figure 4.9), thickening or irregularity of radiating folds, and location on the proximal half of the greater curvature, since benign ulcers are rarely found in this portion of the stomach [21].

Some authors believe that all gastric ulcers should be evaluated by endoscopy and biopsy to rule out gastric carcinoma. However, studies have shown that ulcers with an unequivocally benign appearance on double-contrast examination are invariably benign lesions [20, 21]. In these studies, about two-thirds of all radiographically diagnosed ulcers have had a benign appearance [20, 21]. However, any ulcers with an equivocal or suspicious appearance must be evaluated by endoscopy and biopsy to rule out an ulcerated gastric carcinoma.

No sign in gastrointestinal radiology has generated more confusion than the meniscus sign of a malignant ulcer, originally described by Carman and refined by Kirklin more than 70 years ago [22, 23]. This sign is caused by a cancer straddling

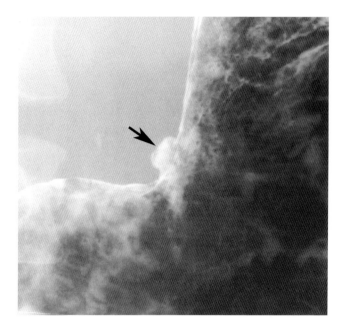

Figure 4.8. Benign gastric ulcer. An ulcer (arrow) is seen projecting beyond the lesser curvature of the gastric body without any associated mass effect. This appearance is characteristic of a benign ulcer viewed in profile.

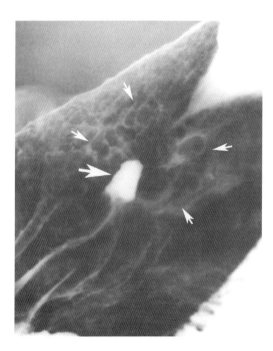

Figure 4.9. Equivocal gastric ulcer. An asymmetric ulcer (large arrow) is seen en face on the posterior wall of the upper gastric body. Note mucosal nodularity and enlarged areae gastricae (small arrows) surrounding the ulcer. This nodularity could be secondary to edema and inflammation versus superficial spread of tumor, so endoscopy is required for a definitive diagnosis. In this case, endoscopic biopsy specimens revealed no evidence of malignant tumor, and the ulcer healed completely on medical treatment with antisecretory agents, so it was a benign gastric ulcer.

the lesser curvature of the gastric antrum or body in which the tumor appears as a broad, flat lesion with central ulceration and elevated margins. Compression of the lesion at fluoroscopy may result in demonstration of a meniscoid ulcer crater that almost always has a convex inner border directed toward the lumen of the stomach and a concave outer border that does not project beyond the expected gastric contour [22, 23]. Although it is thought to be a reliable radiologic sign of malignancy, this sign can be demonstrated in only a small percentage of all patients with malignant ulcers.

Rarely, ulcerated gastric carcinomas involving the greater curvature may spread inferiorly via the gastrocolic ligament to the superior border of the transverse colon, producing a gastrocolic fistula [24]. In today's pill-oriented western society, however, gastrocolic fistulas are more commonly caused by benign greater curvature gastric ulcers due to ingestion of aspirin or other non-steroidal anti-inflammatory drugs (NSAIDs) [25].

Infiltrative carcinomas

Infiltrative carcinomas are circumferential tumors that encase the stomach, causing marked luminal narrowing, often associated with polypoid, ulcerated components and a nodular, spiculated mucosa (Figure 4.10). Eventually, these lesions may cause gastric outlet obstruction. As many as 25% of advanced

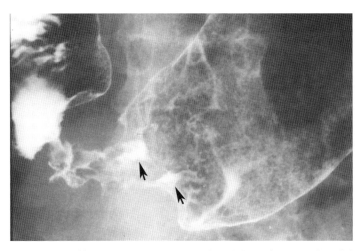

Figure 4.10. Infiltrating gastric carcinoma. There is irregular narrowing of the gastric antrum due to an advanced infiltrating carcinoma. Note areas of ulceration (arrows) within the lesion. Reproduced with permission [13].

carcinomas of the distal antrum involve the duodenum by transpyloric spread of tumor [26]. In such cases, duodenal involvement may be manifested on barium studies by mass effect, nodularity, ulceration, or irregular narrowing of the proximal duodenum.

Scirrhous carcinomas

Scirrhous gastric carcinomas are traditionally thought to arise in the distal stomach, gradually extending from the antrum proximally into the gastric body and fundus (Figure 4.11) [27, 28]. In advanced cases, the entire stomach may be encased by tumor (Figure 4.12). These lesions are classically manifested on barium studies by narrowing and rigidity of the stomach with mucosal nodularity, lobulated folds, and a grossly irregular contour, producing a linitis plastica or "leather bottle" appearance (see Figures 4.11 and 4.12) [27, 28]. This appearance is thought to result pathologically from a marked desmoplastic response incited by the tumor. However, some scirrhous carcinomas may be confined to a relatively short segment of the distal antrum, appearing as annular lesions with shelf-like proximal borders (Figure 4.13) [29]. In such cases, the radiographic findings can sometimes be mistaken for hypertrophic pyloric stenosis.

Despite the classic teaching that scirrhous carcinomas involve the distal half of the stomach, causing marked antral narrowing, it has been found that nearly 40%

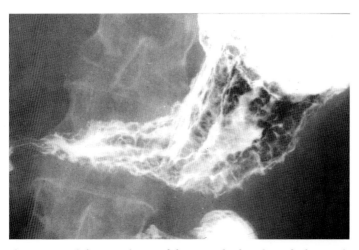

Figure 4.11. Scirrhous carcinoma of the stomach. There is marked narrowing of the gastric antrum and body with considerable nodularity of the mucosa, thickened folds, and an irregular contour, producing a classic linitis plastica appearance.

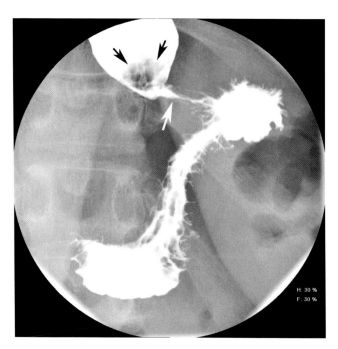

Figure 4.12. Scirrhous carcinoma of the stomach. This patient has diffuse narrowing of the stomach with thickened folds and a grossly irregular contour due to extensive linitis plastica. Note tapered narrowing (white arrow) of the distal esophagus due to tumor invading the gastroesophageal junction, causing secondary achalasia. As a result, there is a bolus of impacted food (black arrows) in the distal esophagus above the narrowed segment.

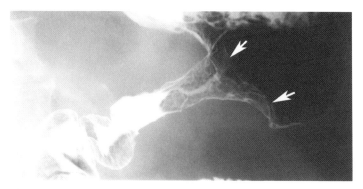

Figure 4.13. Localized scirrhous carcinoma of the distal gastric antrum. There is an annular lesion in the distal gastric antrum. Note how this lesion has an abrupt, shelf-like proximal border (arrows).

of all scirrhous tumors diagnosed on double-contrast studies are confined to the gastric fundus or body with sparing of the antrum (Figure 4.14) [30]. Also, some lesions cause only minimal loss of distensibility in the stomach. Instead, these scirrhous tumors may be recognized on double-contrast studies primarily by distortion of the normal surface pattern of the stomach, with mucosal nodularity, spiculation,

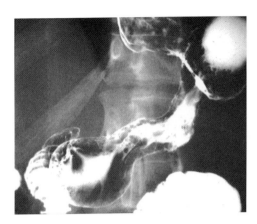

Figure 4.14. Localized scirrhous carcinoma of the gastric body. There is irregular narrowing of the body of the stomach, with sparing of the antrum and fundus. Reproduced with permission [30].

ulceration, and/or thickened, irregular folds [30]. Thus, some lesions are likely to be missed if the radiologist relies too heavily on gastric narrowing as the major criterion for diagnosing these tumors.

It also is important to be aware of the limitations of endoscopy in diagnosing scirrhous carcinomas of the stomach. Because the tumor cells are frequently separated by sheets of fibrosis, endoscopic brushings and biopsy specimens have a sensitivity of less than 50% in detecting these lesions [30, 31, 32]. Thus, multiple endoscopic examinations may be required for a definitive diagnosis, and some patients may even undergo surgery without a preoperative histologic diagnosis.

Although most cases of malignant linitis plastica are caused by primary scirrhous carcinomas, metastatic breast cancer involving the stomach may occasionally produce identical radiographic findings due to a dense infiltrate of metastatic tumor in the gastric wall (Figure 4.15) [30, 33, 34]. The possibility of metastatic disease should therefore be considered in any patient with linitis plastica who has a history of breast cancer.

Non-Hodgkin lymphoma of the stomach is thought to be a rare cause of linitis plastica. It has traditionally been taught that the stomach remains pliable and distensible even when diffusely involved by lymphoma because of the absence of associated fibrosis [35, 36]. In one study, however, it was found that non-Hodgkin lymphoma of the stomach can produce a linitis plastica appearance indistinguishable from that of a scirrhous gastric carcinoma (Figure 4.16) [37]. As in patients with metastatic breast cancer, this finding results pathologically from a dense infiltrate of lymphomatous tissue in the gastric wall [37]. Thus, other malignant tumors should be considered in the differential diagnosis of linitis plastica.

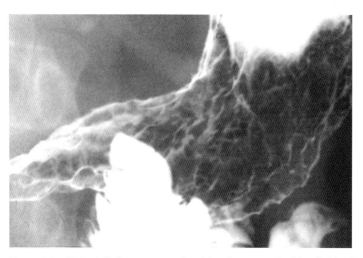

Figure 4.15. Metastatic breast cancer involving the stomach with a linitis plastica appearance. There is narrowing of the gastric antrum and body with considerable nodularity of the overlying mucosa. This appearance is indistinguishable from that of a primary scirrhous carcinoma. Reproduced with permission [30].

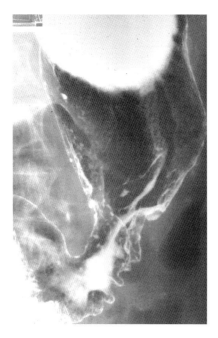

Figure 4.16. Non-Hodgkin lymphoma of the stomach with a linitis plastica appearance. There is narrowing of the lower gastric body with nodularity of the mucosa. This appearance could be mistaken for a primary scirrhous carcinoma of the stomach. Reproduced with permission [37].

Carcinoma of the cardia

The incidence of carcinoma of the cardia has gradually increased since the 1960s; these tumors currently comprise as many as 40% of all gastric cancers [5, 6]. Carcinoma of the cardia has a marked predilection for men (7:1) [3], and a small but significant percentage of patients are under the age of 40 [38]. Radiologists therefore should not be lulled into a false sense of security about the possibility of malignant tumor on the basis of the patient's age. Affected individuals usually present with dysphagia; some patients may have referred dysphagia to the upper chest or even the pharynx. Thus, the gastric cardia and fundus should be carefully evaluated in all patients with dysphagia, regardless of its subjective localization.

Tumors arising at the cardia are notoriously difficult to diagnose on single-contrast barium studies because this area is inaccessible to manual palpation or compression. With the double-contrast technique, however, it is possible to evaluate the normal anatomic landmarks at the cardia and surrounding mucosa for radiographic signs of malignancy. The normal cardia can often be recognized on double-contrast views by three or four stellate folds radiating from a central point at the gastroesophageal junction, also known as the cardiac rosette

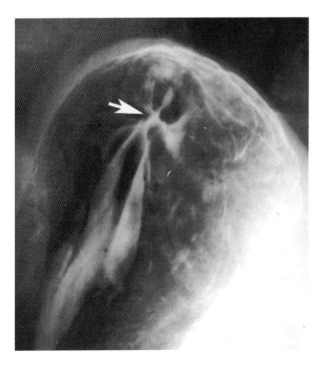

Figure 4.17. Normal gastric cardia. Note folds radiating from a central point (arrow) at the gastroesophageal junction (i.e., the cardiac rosette), best seen on a right-side down, lateral view of the gastric cardia and fundus.

(Figure 4.17) [39, 40]. Some tumors at the cardia may be recognized only by distortion or obliteration of these normal anatomic landmarks, with relatively subtle nodularity, mass effect, and ulceration in this region (Figure 4.18) [39, 40, 41, 42]. Thus, the cardia and fundus should be carefully evaluated by the double-contrast technique in all patients with dysphagia in order to detect these lesions at the earliest possible stage.

Advanced carcinomas of the gastric cardia usually appear on barium studies as polypoid, ulcerated, or infiltrative lesions [41, 43]. Polypoid tumors may be recognized as lobulated or fungating intraluminal masses, often containing irregular areas of ulceration (Figure 4.19). Ulcerated tumors are lesions that have undergone extensive necrosis with a large, irregular area of ulceration in the region of the cardia (Figure 4.20). In contrast, infiltrative lesions may be manifested by thickened, nodular folds and/or decreased distensibility of the fundus due to tumor encasing the gastric wall (Figure 4.21) [42, 43].

Patients with carcinoma of the cardia usually have concomitant esophageal involvement by tumor, manifested by a polypoid mass, thickened folds, or irregular narrowing of the distal esophagus (see Figure 4.18). Submucosal spread of tumor can also result in the development of secondary achalasia, with tapered, beak-like

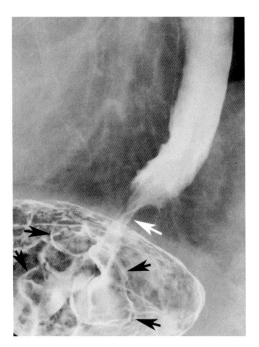

Figure 4.18. Carcinoma of the cardia. There is obliteration of the normal cardiac rosette with irregular areas of mass effect (black arrows) in this region. Also note irregular narrowing (white arrow) of the distal esophagus due to tumor extending across the gastroesophageal junction.

narrowing of the distal esophagus near the gastroesophageal junction (Figures 4.21b and 4.22; also see Figure 4.12) [43, 44]. However, certain morphologic features such as asymmetry, abrupt transitions, and mucosal nodularity or ulceration should suggest an underlying malignancy. Secondary achalasia should also be

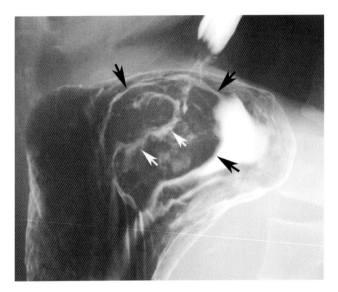

Figure 4.19. Polypoid carcinoma of the cardia. This patient has a polypoid mass (black arrows) that has obliterated and replaced the normal cardiac rosette. Also note areas of ulceration (white arrows) within the mass. Reproduced with permission [19].

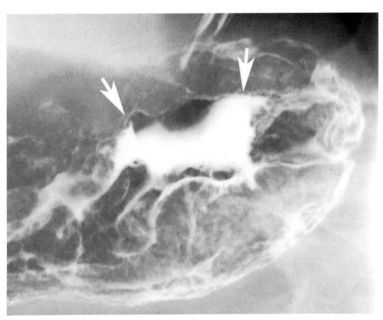

Figure 4.20. Ulcerated carcinoma of the cardia. The cardiac rosette has been obliterated and replaced by an irregular ulcerated lesion (arrows) with thickened, lobulated folds abutting the ulcer.

suspected when the narrowed segment extends proximally a considerable distance from the gastroesophageal junction (see Figure 4.22) [44]. In such cases, careful radiologic evaluation of the fundus is essential to rule out an underlying carcinoma of the cardia as the cause of these findings.

Carcinoma of the cardia invading the esophagus may be indistinguishable on barium studies from a primary esophageal carcinoma invading the gastric cardia [45]. However, cardia carcinomas tend to have a greater degree of gastric involvement in relation to the degree of esophageal involvement, whereas esophageal carcinomas have a greater degree of esophageal involvement. Thus, it is often possible to differentiate between these tumors based on the radiographic findings.

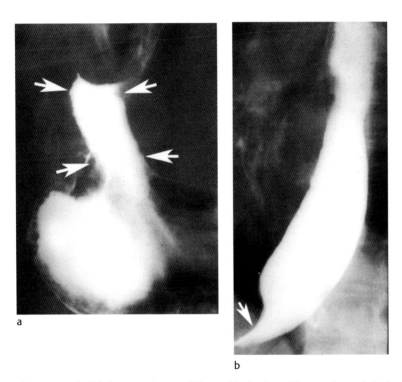

a

b

Figure 4.21a,b. Scirrhous carcinoma of the gastric fundus with secondary achalasia. (a) A view of the fundus shows an advanced scirrhous tumor encasing the proximal stomach (arrows). (b) A view of the esophagus as the patient swallowed barium in the prone, right anterior oblique position shows tapered narrowing (arrow) of the distal esophagus due to tumor invading the gastroesophageal junction. The appearance of the distal esophagus could easily be mistaken for that of primary achalasia.

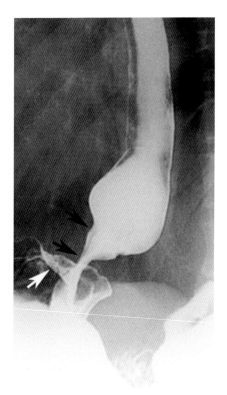

Figure 4.22. Carcinoma of the gastric cardia with secondary achalasia. There is tapered narrowing of the distal esophagus (black arrows), suggesting achalasia. However, a focal area of mass effect (white arrow) is seen in the fundus due to underlying tumor in this region. Also note how the segment of narrowing is longer than that typically seen in patients with primary achalasia.

REFERENCES

1. Devesa SS and Silverman DT. Cancer incidence and mortality trends in the United States: 1935–74. *J Natl Cancer Inst* 1978; **60**: 545–71.

2. Howson CP, Hiyama T, and Wynder EL. The decline in gastric cancer: epidemiology of an unplanned triumph. *Epidemiol Rev* 1986; **8**: 1–27.

3. McBride CM and Boddie AW. Adenocarcinoma of the stomach: are we making any progress? *South Med J* 1987; **80**: 283–6.

4. Cady B, Rossi RL, Silverman ML, Piccione W, and Heck TA. Gastric adenocarcinoma: a disease in transition. *Arch Surg* 1989; **124**: 303–8.

5. Meyers WC, Damiano RJ, Rotolo FS, and Postlethwait RW. Adenocarcinoma of the stomach: changing patterns over the last 4 decades. *Ann Surg* 1987; **205**: 1–8.

6. Antonioli DA and Goldman H. Changes in the location and type of gastric adenocarcinoma. *Cancer* 1982; **50**: 775–81.

7. Kaneko E, Nakamura T, Umeda N, Fujino M, and Niwa H. Outcome of gastric carcinoma detected by gastric mass survey in Japan. *Gut* 1977; **18**: 626–30.

8. Okui K and Tejima H. Evaluation of gastric mass survey. *Acta Chir Scand* 1980; **146**: 185–7.

9. Green PH, O'Toole KM, Slonim D, Wang T, and Weg A. Increasing incidence and excellent survival of patients with early gastric cancer: experience in a United States medical center. *Am J Med* 1988; **85**: 658–61.

10. White RM, Levine MS, Enterline HT, and Laufer I. Early gastric cancer: recent experience. *Radiology* 1985; **155**: 25–7.

11. Murakami T. Pathomorphological diagnosis. In Murakami T ed., *Early Gastric Cancer*. Tokyo: University of Tokyo Press, 1971; pp. 53–5.

12. Levine MS and Laufer I. Tumors of the stomach. In Levine MS, Rubesin SE and Laufer I eds., *Double Contrast Gastrointestinal Radiology*, 3rd edn. Philadelphia, PA: WB Saunders, 2000; pp. 204–38.

13. Levine MS, Megibow AJ, and Kochman ML. Carcinoma of the stomach and duodenum. In Gore RM and Levine MS eds., *Textbook of Gastrointestinal Radiology*, 3rd edn. Philadelphia, PA: WB Saunders, 2008; pp. 619–43.

14. Koga M, Nakata H, Kiyonari H, Inakura M, and Tanaka M. Roentgen features of the superficial depressed type of early gastric carcinoma. *Radiology* 1975; **115**: 289–92.

15. Olearchyk AS. Gastric carcinoma. A critical review of 243 cases. *Am J Gastroenterol* 1978; **70**: 25–45.

16. Thomas RL and Rice RP. Calcifying mucinous adenocarcinoma of the stomach. *Radiology* 1967; **878**: 1002–3.

17. Low VH, Levine MS, Rubesin SE, Laufer I, and Herlinger H. Diagnosis of gastric carcinoma: sensitivity of double-contrast barium studies. *AJR Am J Roentgenol* 1994; **162**: 329–34.

18. Wolf BS. Observations on roentgen features of benign and malignant gastric ulcers. *Semin Roentgenol* 1971; **6**: 140–50.

19. Rubesin SE, Levine MS, and Laufer I. Double-contrast upper gastrointestinal radiography: a pattern approach for diseases of the stomach. *Radiology* 2008; **246**: 33–48.

20. Thompson G, Somers S, and Stevenson GW. Benign gastric ulcer: a reliable radiologic diagnosis? *AJR Am J Roentgenol* 1983; **141**: 331–3.

21. Levine MS, Creteur V, Kressel HY, Laufer I, and Herlinger H. Benign gastric ulcers: diagnosis and follow-up with double-contrast radiography. *Radiology* 1987; **164**: 9–13.

22. Carman RD. A new roentgen-ray sign of ulcerating gastric cancer. *J Am Med Assoc* 1921; **77**: 990–2.

23. Kirklin BR. The value of the meniscus sign in the roentgenologic diagnosis of ulcerating gastric carcinoma. *Radiology* 1934; **22**: 131–5.

24. Smith DL, Dockerty MB, and Black BM. Gastrocolic fistulas of malignant origin. *Surg Gynecol Obstet* 1972; **134**: 829–32.

25. Levine MS, Kelly MR, Laufer I, Rubesin SE, and Herlinger H. Gastrocolic fistulas: the increasing role of aspirin. *Radiology* 1993; **187**: 359–61.

26. Cho KC, Baker SR, Alterman DD, Fusco JM, and Cho S. Transpyloric spread of gastric tumors: comparison of adenocarcinoma and lymphoma. *AJR Am J Roentgenol* 1996; **167**: 467–9.

27. Raskin MM. Some specific radiological findings and consideration of linitis plastica of the gastrointestinal tract. *CRC Crit Rev Clin Radiol Nucl Med* 1976; **8**: 87–106.

28. Marshak RH, Lindner AE, and Maklansky D. Carcinoma of the stomach. In Marshak RH, Lindner AE and Maklansky D eds., *Radiology of the Stomach*. Philadelphia, PA: WB Saunders, 1983; pp. 108–46.

29. Balthazar EJ, Rosenberg H, and Davidian MM. Scirrhous carcinoma of the pyloric channel and distal antrum. *AJR Am J Roentgenol* 1980; **134**: 669–73.

30. Levine MS, Kong V, Rubesin SE, Laufer I, and Herlinger H. Scirrhous carcinoma of the stomach: radiologic and endoscopic diagnosis. *Radiology* 1990; **175**: 151–4.

31. Winawer SJ, Posner G, Lightdale CJ, Sherlock P, Melamed M, and Fortner JG. Endoscopic diagnosis of advanced gastric cancer. Factors influencing yield. *Gastroenterology* 1975; **69**: 1183–7.

32. Evans E, Harris O, Dickey D, and Hartley L. Difficulties in the endoscopic diagnosis of gastric and oesophageal cancer. *Aust N Z J Surg* 1985; **55**: 541–4.

33. Joffe N. Metastatic involvement of the stomach secondary to breast carcinoma. *AJR Am J Roentgenol* 1975; **123**: 512–21.

34. Cormier WJ, Gaffey TA, Welch JM, Welch JS, and Edmonson JH. Linitis plastica caused by metastatic lobular carcinoma of the breast. *Mayo Clin Proc* 1980; **55**: 747–53.

35. Sherrick DW, Hodgson JR, and Dockerty MB. The roentgenologic diagnosis of primary gastric lymphoma. *Radiology* 1965; **84**: 925–32.

36. Menuck LS. Gastric lymphoma: a radiologic diagnosis. *Gastrointest Radiol* 1976; **1**: 157–61.

37. Levine MS, Pantongrag-Brown L, Aguilera NS, Buck JL and Buetow PC. Non-Hodgkin lymphoma of the stomach: a cause of linitis plastica. *Radiology* 1996; **201**: 375–8.

38. MacDonald WC. Clinical and pathologic features of adenocarcinoma of the gastric cardia. *Cancer* 1972; **29**: 724–32.

39. Freeny PC. Double-contrast gastrography of the fundus and cardia: normal landmarks and their pathologic changes. *AJR Am J Roentgenol* 1979; **133**: 481–7.

40. Herlinger H, Grossman R, Laufer I, Kressel HY, and Ochs RH. The gastric cardia in double-contrast study: its dynamic image. *AJR Am J Roentgenol* 1980; **135**: 21–9.

41. Freeny PC and Marks WM. Adenocarcinoma of the gastroesophageal junction: barium and CT examination. *AJR Am J Roentgenol* 1982; **138**: 1077–84.

42. Levine MS, Laufer I, and Thompson JJ. Carcinoma of the gastric cardia in young people. *AJR Am J Roentgenol* 1983; **140**: 69–72.

43. Balthazar EJ, Goldfine S, and Davidian MM. Carcinoma of the esophagogastric junction. *Am J Gastroenterol* 1980; **74**: 237–43.

44. Woodfield CA, Levine MS, Rubesin SE, Langlotz CP, and Laufer I. Diagnosis of primary versus secondary achalasia: reassessment of clinical and radiographic criteria. *AJR Am J Roentgenol* 2000; **175**: 727–31.

45. Levine MS, Caroline DF, Thompson JJ, Kressel HY, Laufer I, and Herlinger H. Adenocarcinoma of the esophagus: relationship to Barrett mucosa. *Radiology* 1984; **150**: 305–9.

5

Surgical management of gastric cancer

Marshall S. Baker, Mark S. Talamonti, and Malcolm M. Bilimoria

Epidemiology

Although the incidence of esophageal adenocarcinoma and gastroesophageal junction malignancies is increasing, by all measures, the incidence of true gastric cancers appears to be in decline. Even through the late 1990s, stomach cancer was the second most common cancer worldwide. In 2008 there were an estimated 974 000 new cases/year. In 2008, the age-adjusted incidence of gastric cancer was about 15% less than that for 1985 [1]. Nonetheless, gastric cancer remains a leading cause of morbidity and mortality, particularly in Asia.

Pathology and staging

The most commonly used staging system is that approved by the American Joint Committee on Cancer and the International Union Against Cancer (Table 5.1) [2]. This system classifies lesions on the basis of the depth of invasion of the gastric wall, the number of regional lymph nodes involved, and the presence or absence of distant metastasis. The staging system is discussed in Chapter 7.

Neoadjuvant therapy

One of the more important developments in the treatment of gastric cancer has been the demonstration of the clinical efficacy in a large randomized trial studying preoperative chemoradiation. For several decades chemotherapy has been an accepted part of the treatment in patients with advanced gastric cancer (AGC), with multiple prior studies demonstrating a survival advantage over surgery alone [3]. Prior to 2006 there had been no level-one evidence to support the efficacy of using chemotherapy in a neoadjuvant setting in the management of gastric

Table 5.1. American Joint Committee on Cancer
Staging System for Gastric Carcinoma [2]

Stage	T	N	M
Stage 0	Tis	N0	M0
Stage IA	T1	N0	M0
Stage IB	T1	N1	M0
	T2a, T2b	N0	M0
Stage II	T1	N2	M0
	T2a, T2b	N1	M0
	T3	N0	M0
Stage IIIA	T2a, T2b	N2	M0
	T3	N1	M0
	T4	N0	M0
Stage IIIB	T3	N2	M0
Stage IV	T4	N1, N2, N3	M0
	T1, T2, T3	N3	M0
	Any T	Any N	M1

adenocarcinoma. The multi-institutional Medical Research Council Adjuvant Gastric Infusional Chemotherapy (MAGIC) trial conducted in the United Kingdom and the Netherlands randomized patients with resectable (determined by preoperative CT imaging, by endoscopic ultrasound or both) adenocarcinoma of the stomach and gastroesophageal junction to either perioperative chemotherapy with epirubicin, cisplatin and fluorouracil (ECF) and subsequent resection or surgery alone. Perioperative chemotherapy consisted of three cycles preoperatively and three cycles postoperatively. Epirubicin and cisplatin were given intravenously on the first day of each cycle and fluorouracil was given daily for 21 days as a continuous infusion therapy. The trial allowed for dose modification based on side-effects. Patients were followed for a median of 50 months after therapy. Patients in either arm had similar rates of perioperative morbidity but patients receiving perioperative ECF demonstrated a statistically significant survival benefit, with an overall 5-year survival in the ECF group of 36% compared to 23% for the group that was randomized to surgery alone. This important trial has laid the foundation for the use of preoperative chemotherapy in an effort to down-size gastric cancers prior to surgical resection [4]. The group treated with perioperative ECF did indeed demonstrate morbidity related to the chemotherapy: 90% of patients had a grade 0, 1 or 2 adverse reaction. A sizeable minority of patients had a grade 3 or 4 reaction. These side-effects included both hematologic (leukopenia) and non-hematologic side-effects (nausea, diarrhea, neurologic). Of 215 patients, 6 did not go on to receive surgery following the preoperative chemotherapy and only 42% of patients randomized to the perioperative chemotherapy arm actually completed all pre- and postoperative therapy. Despite the low completion rates, a benefit was seen for all patients enrolled. Clearly, for patients with a marginal functional status prior to therapy, consideration should be given to the impact that preoperative chemotherapy may have on the ability of the patient to tolerate resection. This is particularly important in light of the significant nutritional depletion that many of these patients have experienced by the time of diagnosis. Ideally, each patient with gastric cancer should be presented to medical oncology in the form of a multidisciplinary gastrointestinal (GI) tumor board for consideration of neoadjuvant therapy.

Surgical therapy for gastric cancer

Over the last decade, extensive investigation by groups of medical oncologists and GI surgeons has been dedicated to improving the surgical care of patients with gastric adenocarcinoma. Specifically, these efforts have been dedicated to defining the extent of surgical resection (Figure 5.1), the efficacy of laparoscopic surgical resection, and the extent of the perigastric lymphadenectomy (Figure 5.2). We will review the literature that has been developed in these areas before proceeding with a description of our surgical approach (Figure 5.3) to the patient with gastric cancer.

Extent of resection

In the latter part of the twentieth century, there continued to be debate over the required extent of gastric resection even in regard to the treatment of antral tumors. A number of groups both in the United States and abroad felt strongly that either a near-total or total gastrectomy was required to adequately treat these cancers. In an effort to resolve this issue several groups initiated randomized trials comparing total gastrectomy with partial gastrectomy with 6-cm gross margins. Uniformly these studies have demonstrated that both disease-free and overall survival rates are similar for total gastrectomy compared with distal or subtotal gastrectomy. The most notable of these studies is an Italian multi-institutional randomized trial involving 28 centers and comparing total with partial gastrectomy in 600 patients followed for 5 years. This study demonstrated overall survival rates of 64% at 5 years for both groups [5]. Additional retrospective and prospective studies have shown shorter

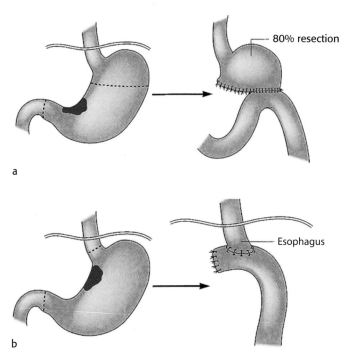

80% resection

Esophagus

a

b

Figure 5.1a–c. Standard open operations for advanced gastric carcinoma. At the present time, surgical extirpation is the only method of cure for invasive gastric cancer. (a) For distal cancers, a subtotal gastrectomy with gastrojejunal reconstruction is performed. (b) For invasive cancers of the gastric body, total gastrectomy with esophagojejunostomy is indicated. (c) Cancers of the proximal stomach are treated with esophagogastrectomy with anastomosis in a cervical or thoracic position. From Mercer DW, Robinson EK. Stomach. In Townsend CM, Beauchamp RD, Evers BM and Mattox KL eds., *Sabiston Textbook of Surgery***, 18th edn. Philadelphia, PA: WB Saunders, 2007; Figure 48.12, p. 750.**

lengths of stay and improved postoperative oral intake, nutrition, and functional health in subtotal resection.

Given these findings, we strongly believe that extent of resection should be determined by the location of the tumor. Proximal tumors may require a near-total gastrectomy to achieve adequate margins, but distal, antral, and body tumors are best managed with partial gastrectomies with an effort to preserve as much of a remnant stomach as possible.

Laparoscopic approaches

With the advent of laparoscopic cholecystectomy in the early 1990s a strong interest in developing minimally invasive approaches to surgical management of GI

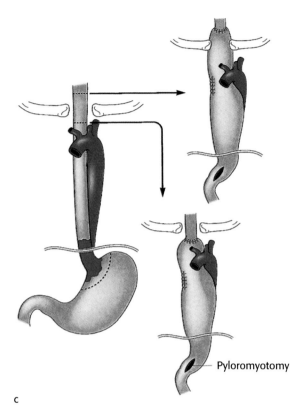

c

Figure 5.1. (Cont.)

neoplasia has emerged. These have included the early development of laparoscopic colectomy and hepatectomy for malignant disease and laparoscopic pancreatectomy for premalignant cystic pancreatic disease. Laparoscopic gastrectomy has been relatively slow to evolve primarily because of concern over the ability of the laparoscopic approach to provide an adequate lymphadenectomy.

There have been several substantial efforts to apply laparoscopic techniques to gastric adenocarcinoma with curative intent [6, 7]. One large retrospective review in Japan examined outcomes following laparoscopic gastrectomy (distal and subtotal) in the management of 1294 patients with early stage gastric cancer (Stage I or II). This review demonstrated very good outcomes for these individuals, with perioperative morbidity of less than 15% and 5-year disease-free survival of greater than 85% [6]. There has been at least one small randomized trial comparing laparoscopic to open gastrectomy for gastric adenocarcinoma. This was a single-institution Italian study that randomly assigned 59 patients with resectable gastric adenocarcinoma to either

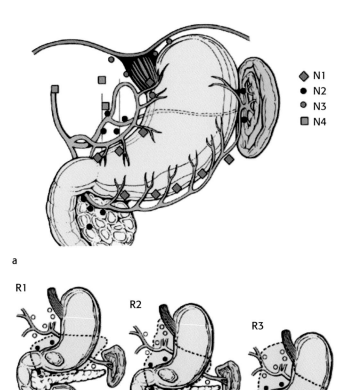

◆ N1
● N2
◯ N3
▢ N4

a

b

Figure 5.2a,b. Level of lymph node dissection. Data from several series suggest that the level of lymph node dissection accompanying gastrectomy for gastric cancer can influence survival. The lymphadenectomies that have come into use are classified according to the specific echelon of nodes removed and may differ depending on tumor location. (a) Tiers of nodes from perigastric (N1) to para-aortic (N4) are shown. (b) Removal of the primary draining lymph nodes (N1), shown as closed circles, with greater and lesser omenta is an R1 dissection and constitutes the minimal acceptable operation for gastric cancer. R2 dissection requires secondary lymph node excision (N2) in the celiac and hepatic regions, as well as splenic hilar nodes when the tumor involves the adjacent stomach. Splenectomy is controversial as a means of removing the latter nodes. More extensive dissections (R3) of tertiary nodes and the lining of the lesser sac are rarely performed because of their greater morbidity and unclear benefits.

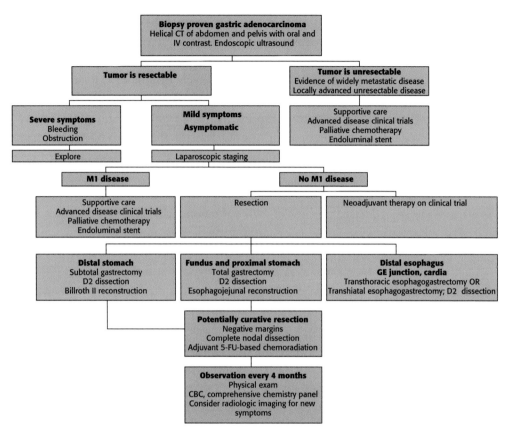

Figure 5.3. Algorithm highlighting surgical approach to the patient with gastric cancer.

laparoscopic or open gastrectomy. The preoperative demographics were similar across groups and the patients were followed for a median of 5 years. The average number of lymph nodes excised was comparable at a mean of 30 lymph nodes resected by each method. The perioperative morbidity rates were statistically identical at close to 27% and the actuarial survival was also comparable, with both groups demonstrating 5-year disease-free survival of 55% [7]. This evidence confirms the efficacy of laparoscopic resection by surgeons with significant experience of laparoscopic gastrectomy. The majority of gastric resections, however, continue to be done in an open fashion.

Staging laparoscopy

There have been several studies investigating preoperative diagnostic laparoscopy as a tool for the management of patients with gastric cancer. Each of these has demonstrated the ability of simple diagnostic laparoscopy to detect the presence of M1 disease that was not evident on preoperative staging imaging. Some of these studies include peritoneal washings to help determine subsequent therapy. The exact rate at which preoperative laparoscopy detects distant disease and changes the management of the patients varies from 15% to 50% [8, 9, 10].

A recent study utilizing current multidetector CT (MDCT) imaging technology performed diagnostic laparoscopy on 71 patients thought to have potentially resectable disease on preoperative imaging studies. Sixteen (23%) of these patients were found to have distant metastasis as evidenced by metastatic nodules in the liver or peritoneal carcinomatosis. In 12 of the patients a laparotomy was avoided [9]; 4 of the 16 underwent laparotomy for palliation.

Current studies evaluating preoperative laparoscopy are limited in two fundamental ways. First, most of these series do not segregate the cases on the basis of final staging pathology. Clearly early-stage (T1 and T2) tumors are less likely to have peritoneal disease at the time of resection, making diagnostic laparoscopy less useful. The data currently do not allow us to draw a conclusion about the utility of diagnostic laparoscopy in early-stage gastric cancer. Secondly, it is unclear whether diagnostic laparoscopy is effective in ultimately changing management when done prior to neoadjuvant therapy for gastric cancer. Generally our approach is to perform pretreatment laparoscopy in patients prior to neoadjuvant therapy only if there is evidence on preoperative imaging (ascites or omental caking on CT) that the patient is not amenable for whatever reason to evaluation by endoscopic ultrasound or CT-guided biopsy.

There are several small studies that evaluate the ability of peritoneal washing and cytology to detect cancer cells in early and late T-stage tumors. There is a significant rate of positive cytology in tumors that are T3 and T4, however there is no evidence to suggest that peritoneal cytology is effective in changing the pre-resection stage of the disease or that peritoneal washings add any additional information to that provided by simple diagnostic laparoscopy alone [10].

Lymphadenectomy

The extent of lymph node dissection required for adequate treatment of gastric cancer has been a topic of extensive debate and repeated evaluation. In general, Japanese surgeons have widely favored and strongly lobbied for extended lymphadenectomies in the treatment of gastric cancer. The extent of these lymphadenectomies is dependent on the location of the tumors but typically includes omentectomy with resection of the anterior leaflet of the transverse mesocolon and resections of nodal basins around the celiac axis, hepatic artery, and left gastric artery.

For proximal gastric cancers a distal pancreatectomy and splenectomy are performed to clear the peripancreatic and perisplenic lymph nodes. This component of the resection has been called a D2 lymphadenectomy. Western surgeons have generally preferred less extensive lymph node resections, limiting their lymphadenectomies to a resection of the gastrocolic omentum, along with the retropyloric and perigastric lymph nodes within 3 cm of the tumor (D1 lymphadenectomy). Still others have advocated a modified D2 resection including the gastrocolic omentum, perigastric nodes and nodes along the celiac axis, left gastric artery and hepatic artery, but not the anterior leaflet of the transverse mesocolon or the nodes at the hilum of the spleen.

There have been two large prospective randomized trials designed to compare the survival outcomes following D1 and D2 lymphadenectomy for gastric cancers, one done in the United Kingdom and a more recent trial from the Netherlands. In the Dutch trial, patients with resectable gastric cancers were randomly assigned to undergo either a D2 or a D1 dissection. The lymph node resections were done by a select group of Dutch surgeons who had been specially trained by experienced gastric cancer surgeons from Japan. Each surgery was overseen by an experienced gastric surgeon to be sure that the assigned lymphadenectomy was being performed appropriately. Splenectomy in both groups was left to the discretion of the surgeon. Median follow-up was 5 years for both groups. The results of this trial demonstrated a higher rate of perioperative complications in the D2 group and statistically identical rates of disease-free survival. Much of the postoperative morbidity and mortality in the group undergoing the more extensive D2 dissection came as a result of postoperative pancreatic fistulae associated simply with the pancreatectomy done in the D2 dissection [11]. Nonetheless the finding that the rates of disease-free survival are comparable has led most gastric cancer surgeons to favor a more limited lymphadenectomy. Similarly, the UK study showed equivalent long-term survival for patients undergoing either the D1 or the D2 lymphadenectomy although this study did not have the same oversight by Japanese gastric surgeons [12].

The current AJCC staging system does stage patients on the basis of the number of nodes that are positive and not on the level of lymph nodes resected (D1 versus D2). The number of lymph nodes examined is important for providing prognostic information to gastric cancer patients. Karpeh and colleagues recently reviewed the experience at the Memorial Sloan Kettering Cancer Center from 1985 to 1999. In this series, 1038 patient cases were reviewed retrospectively. The authors found that disease-free survival was statistically better for patients who had more than 15 lymph nodes examined pathologically when compared stage for stage with patients who had fewer than 15 lymph nodes examined. This result likely reflects an under-staging phenomenon in the latter group but does support the notion that the number of nodes resected is important in providing accurate prognostic information using the current AJCC system [13].

Our preoperative evaluation

Endoscopic ultrasound has become increasingly important in the preoperative staging of gastric cancer patients. This test provides accurate determination of the depth of mural invasion by the tumor and, in some instances, the cytologic evaluation of the lymph nodes in the celiac, hepatic artery, and retropancreatic basins. There is no level-one evidence to demonstrate a benefit of the use of endoscopic ultrasound in the preoperative evaluation of patients with gastric cancer; however, our routine is for all patients with potentially resectable gastric malignancy to have a chest radiograph, high-quality triphasic abdominal CT scan, and endoscopic ultrasonography (EUS) evaluation prior to surgery. Tumor marker serologies (carcinoembryonic antigen or CEA) are also routine. Each patient is then presented preoperatively at our Multidisciplinary Gastrointestinal Tumor Board. During this discussion, the group designs an individualized treatment plan utilizing neoadjuvant therapy where appropriate depending on the functional status of the patient and the preoperative stage of the tumor.

Our preferred surgical technique – distal tumors

In general, we use exploratory laparoscopy (Figure 5.4) to initiate any gastric cancer surgery. This is done with two trocars. One is a supraumbilical trocar that is placed via a Hasson technique while the other is typically placed in the left mid abdomen. In our minds the Hasson technique minimizes any potential for vascular and intestinal injury that might be incurred using a Verres needle. A 30° side-viewing camera is inserted through the umbilical port and used to inspect the abdomen. A blunt grasper is placed through the 5-mm port and used to manipulate the bowel. Using these instruments a thorough laparoscopic exploration is performed. We generally survey the four quadrants of the abdomen for ascites and carcinomatosis (see Figure 5.4) that may be on the peritoneal surfaces. Any suspicious nodules are biopsied and any ascites sent for cytologic examination. The transverse colon

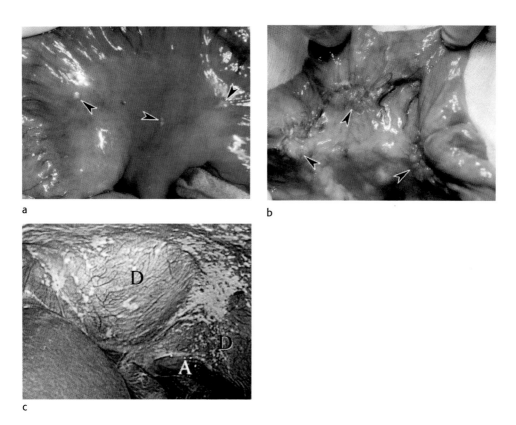

Figure 5.4a–c. Staging laparoscopy: intraoperative images. Small mesenteric implants (arrowheads) are seen in (a) and (b), which confirmed the presence of M1 disease in these patients with negative CT scans. (c) Metastatic implants presenting as whitish plaques are seen on the serosal aspect of the duodenum (D). A, Ascites.

is retracted upward and the root of the mesentery is also inspected for peritoneal nodularity. The gastrocolic omentum is opened and the lesser sac accessed. This location posterior to the proximal stomach is an area where low-volume carcinomatosis is encountered.

We are not yet convinced that our lymphadenectomy done laparoscopically is comparable to that which we perform via an open surgical technique. As a result, we do not routinely do laparoscopic gastrectomy for gastric cancer. If there are no abnormal findings on the diagnostic laparoscopy, the laparoscope is withdrawn and an upper abdominal incision is created. The first steps following this are performed to confirm the findings at laparoscopy through open examination of the abdomen. The stomach is manually palpated. The tumor is identified and confirmed to be free of any direct extension into the retroperitoneum below. The liver is manually inspected and lesions that raise suspicion of metastatic disease are biopsied. An intraoperative ultrasound can be useful as part of the evaluation of the liver. This is particularly true if the preoperative axial CT images have demonstrated small but questionable lesions in the liver.

The duodenum is mobilized from the retroperitoneum by means of a Kocher maneuver and the lymph nodes between the aorta and the inferior vena cava are inspected manually. Any nodes in this location that are felt to be pathologically enlarged are sent for frozen section examination. Nodes in this area or nodules in the liver that are positive on frozen section generally preclude any possibility of an R0 resection (i.e., complete surgical extirpation of tumor) and the operation is terminated.

Once this examination is completed and resectability confirmed, we proceed with the formal steps of the resection. The tumor is again localized and its position relative to the left gastric artery and the short gastric vessels noted. For distal tumors a proximal margin of at least 6 cm is marked. The gastrocolic ligament is taken along the border of the colon along the entire length of the transverse colon. This allows the omentum to be taken en bloc with the specimen. The splenic flexure of the colon is routinely mobilized to avoid injury to the inferior pole of the spleen with retraction. The short gastric vessels are also taken, usually using a bipolar cautery device. In the case of distal tumors the short gastric ligation continues up to the level of the stomach, which has been identified as the proximal margin of resection.

The gastrohepatic ligament is then taken close to the undersurface of the left lateral segment of the liver. The left gastric artery is routinely preserved as part of a distal gastrectomy. The lymph node basin along the border of the proper hepatic artery, left gastric artery, and over the celiac axis is removed en bloc with the resection specimen. The right gastroepiploic artery and vein are ligated via sutures at their origin over the neck of the pancreas. The gastropancreatic fold is divided and the pylorus liberated from the neck of the pancreas. The specimen is then removed using a GI stapler. The stapler is used to divide the duodenum approximately 2 cm distal to the pylorus. Achieving this distance is imperative in an effort to provide an adequate margin on the tumor and to avoid postoperative complications from retained antral mucosa. The stapling device is used to divide the stomach at a location that is again confirmed to be at least 6 cm proximal to the tumor. The distal and proximal margins are marked and the entire specimen including the omentum, celiac lymph node packet, and stomach is submitted to pathology. Frozen sections are sent to confirm clear proximal and distal margins.

The reconstruction in a distal resection begins with the oversewing of the gastric and duodenal remnants. This is done with interrupted silk sutures in a Lembert fashion. A Roux limb is then created by dividing the jejunum approximately 20 cm distal to the ligament of Treitz. The distal Roux limb is brought up to the gastric remnant in a retrocolic fashion to the left of the middle colic vessels. The staple line at the cut end of this limb is oversewn with silk Lembert sutures. The gastrojejunal anastomosis is made to the posterior wall of the gastric remnant in a side-to-side functional end-to-end isoperistaltic fashion. This is either handsewn using two layers of suture (an inner layer of absorbable Vicryl and an outer layer of non-absorbable silk suture) or constructed using a GI stapler.

Our preferred surgical technique – proximal tumors

For proximal tumors, a total or subtotal gastrectomy is performed. These resections begin with a thorough exploration via an upper midline incision as in the case of the distal tumor. The beginning of the resection proceeds in essentially the same manner as for distal tumors. For proximal tumors, all short gastric vessels are taken to the level of the esophagus. The entire gastrocolic omentum is resected. The left gastric artery is also routinely divided at its origin. GI continuity is again re-established using a Roux limb. This limb is made to be 60 cm in distance between the esophagojejunostomy and the duodenojejunostomy in an effort to avoid reflux of bile into the distal esophagus. A "J" pouch is constructed in the Roux limb at the site of the esophagojejunostomy. This is done by folding the jejunum back on itself for a length of approximately 20 cm and a long jejunojejunostomy is created using a GI stapler. An esophagojejunostomy is then fashioned between the bend in this segment and the distal esophagus using either a handsewn or a stapled technique. A feeding jejunostomy is routinely placed at the end of all total gastrectomies.

Outcomes

Gastric cancer continues to be a substantial source of mortality. In the most recent Memorial review, the 5-year disease-specific survival for resected patients was 49%. Predictors of survival in a multivariate analysis include depth of invasion, number of positive lymph nodes (N stage), and tumor site. Looking just at patients who had positive lymph nodes, the overall disease-specific survival was 27% for 5 years [13]. The importance of the number of positive lymph nodes as a predictor of outcome has been corroborated by several large series [14, 15]. These data are summarized in Table 5.2.

Table 5.2. Survival after curative resection of gastric cancer according to lymph node status

Lymph node status	Roder [14]		Kodera et al. [15]		Karpeh et al. [13]	
	Cases	5-year Survival (%)	Cases	5-year Survival (%)	Cases	5-year Survival (%)
N1 (1–6 positive nodes)	258	45	306	70	392	38
N2 (7–15 positive nodes)	137	30	94	39	178	12
N3 (> 15 positive nodes)	82	10	93	24	65	5

Conclusions

Surgical resection is the only effective treatment for advanced gastric cancers. Preoperative staging can spare many patients an unnecessary operation but most patients will come for exploratory laparotomy. The aim of a stage-appropriate operation for gastric cancer must be to apply a treatment designed for maximum survival time while allowing the patient to enjoy an optimal quality of life. Advances in diagnostic and therapeutic laparoscopic procedures for the patient with gastric cancer should help optimize patient management [16].

REFERENCES

1. Brenner H, Rothenbacher D, and Arndt V. Epidemiology of stomach cancer. *Methods Mol Biol* 2009; **472**: 467–77.
2. Greene FL, Page DL, Balch CM, Fleming ID, and Morrow M eds. Stomach. In *AJCC Cancer Staging Manual*, 6th edn. New York, NY: Springer, 2002; pp. 99–106.
3. Van De Velde CJH. Current role of surgery and multimodal treatment in localized gastric cancer. *Ann Oncol* 2008; **19**: 93–8.
4. Cunningham D, Allum WH, Stenning SP *et al.* Perioperative chemotherapy versus surgery alone for resectable gastroesophageal cancer. *N Engl J Med* 2006; **355**: 11–20.
5. Bozzetti F, Marubini E, Bonfanti G, Miceli R, Piano C, and Gennari L. Subtotal versus total gastrectomy for gastric cancer. *Ann Surg* 1999; **230**: 170–8.
6. Kitano S, Shiraishi N, Uyama I, Sugihara K, and Tanigawa N. A multicenter study on oncologic outcome of laparoscopic gastrectomy for early cancer in Japan. *Ann Surg* 2007; **245**: 68–72.

7. Huscher CGS, Mingoli A, Sgarzini G *et al.* Laparoscopic versus open subtotal gastrectomy for distal gastric cancer; five year results of a randomized prospective trial. *Ann Surg* 2005; **241**: 232–7.

8. Possik RA, Franco EL, and Pires DR. Sensitivity, specificity and predictive value of laparoscopy for the staging of gastric cancer and for the detection of liver metastases. *Cancer* 1986; **58**: 1–6.

9. Kriplani AK and Kapur BML. Laparoscopy for pre-operative staging and assessment of operability in gastric carcinoma. *Gastrointest Endosc* 1991; **37**: 441–3.

10. Lowy AM, Mansfield PF, and Steven D. Laparoscopic staging for gastric cancer. *Surgery* 1996; **119**: 611–14.

11. Bonenkamp JJ, Hermans J, Sasako M, and Van De Velde CJH. Extended lymph-node dissection for gastric cancer. *New Engl J Med* 1999; **340**: 908–14.

12. Cuschieri A, Weeden S, Fielding J *et al.* Patient survival after D1 and D2 resections for gastric cancer: long-term results of the MRC randomized surgical trial. *Br J Can* 1999; **79**: 1522–30.

13. Karpeh MS, Leon L, Klimstra D, and Brenan MF. Lymph node staging in gastric cancer: is location more important than number? *Ann Surg* 2000; **3**: 362–71.

14. Roder DM. The epidemiology of gastric caner. *Gastric Cancer* 2002; **5**(1): 5–11.

15. Kodera Y, Yamamura Y, and Shimizu Y. Lymph node status assessment for gastric carcinoma: is the number of metastatic lymph nodes really practical as a parameter for N category in the TNM classification? Tumor node metastasis. *J Surg Oncol* 1998; **69**(1): 15–20.

16. Yoo CH, Kim HO, Hwang SI *et al.* Short-term outcomes of laparoscopic-assisted distal gastrectomy for gastric cancer during a surgeon's learning curve period. *Surg Endosc* 2009; Jan 27. (Epub ahead of print.)

6

Systemic therapy for gastric cancer

Janardan D. Khandekar and Melin Khandekar

Introduction

Gastric cancer was the leading cause of cancer-related death worldwide through-out most of the twentieth century, and now ranks second only to lung cancer, with an estimated 950 000 new cases diagnosed annually [1]. The incidence of gastric cancer varies widely in different countries. In the United States, the incidence has dramatically decreased, and in the year 2009, 21 600 new cases are expected to be diagnosed [1]. One of the most important factors implicated in the pathogenesis of gastric cancer is infection with *Helicobacter pylori*. Studies have shown that this organism is especially adaptable in the hostile gastric environment. An antigen known as CagA, a 120- to 130-kDa protein encoded by *cagA* genes of *H. pylori*, interacts directly with host epithelial cells, causing epithelial cell proliferation and ultimately benign gastritis. In more severe cases, a phenotype termed the "gastric cancer phenotype" develops, which is characterized by a predominant pattern of gastritis in the body of the stomach with gastric atrophy and hypochlorhydria. Correa has described in detail the multi-step multifactorial process in the genesis of gastric cancer [2, 3].

While *H. pylori* infection is very prevalent, far fewer than 1% of infected indi-viduals will develop gastric cancer. Previous studies have linked *H. pylori* infection to the overexpression of interleukin-1β (IL-1β). Recent studies using a transgenic mouse model show that IL-1β works by activating myeloid-derived suppressor cells, which are strongly pro-inflammatory. Blocking IL-1β or the myeloid-derived suppressor cells may be a potential strategy for preventing gastric cancer.

Early gastric cancer (EGC) is an adenocarcinoma confined to the mucosa with or without lymph node metastasis. In Japan, EGCs account for approximately 50% of all newly diagnosed cancer, while in Western countries they account for only 15%–20% [4, 5]. About 5% of gastric carcinomas may be squamous or adenosquamous cell type, and rarely small cell carcinomas have also been detected. These small cell carcinomas respond to chemotherapy in a very similar way to small cell cancer of the lung [6].

One of the most striking epidemiologic observations in recent years has been the increasing incidence of adenocarcinoma involving the distal esophagus and proximal stomach. A meta-analysis by Islami and Kamangar [7] showed that there is an inverse association between CagA-positive *H. pylori* colonization and the risk of gastric adenocarcinoma. Thus, the decline of *H. pylori* in the United States from over 70% in the early 1960s to about 9% currently may be partly responsible for the decreased incidence of gastric carcinoma, but an increased incidence in gastroesophageal junction tumors. These epidemiologic observations have implications for the systemic therapy of gastric cancer.

Patterns of metastases

The treatment of gastric cancer is governed by patterns of regional and distant failure. Carcinoma of the stomach can spread by local extension and involve adjacent structures or it can develop lymphatic, peritoneal, or hematogenous metastasis. Both anatomic and biologic factors determine the wide variations in patterns of metastases.

In the West, gastric cancers often present in more advanced stages, and in large studies 60% of resected gastric patients have evidence of serosal involvement while in 68% lymph nodes contain cancer [5, 8]. The apparent patterns of metastases have changed due to the use of different treatment modalities and through newer imaging modalities (see Chapter 7). Endoscopic ultrasound is an important tool for staging EGC. Computed tomography (CT) and magnetic resonance imaging (MRI) also play an important role [9]. Recent studies have observed that in patients whose disease recurs, local/regional metastases are found in over 50%, while 30% of patients who recur have peritoneal metastases. Distant metastases also occur in a significant proportion of patients depending on the stage of gastric cancer. These and other studies serve to identify patterns of metastasis and thus formulate strategy for adjuvant treatment approaches.

Systemic therapy

In comparing the results of systemic therapy of cancer, it is important to keep in mind the staging of gastric cancer. The American Joint Commission on Cancer Staging/UICC TNM Staging for Gastric Cancer is shown as Table 6.1 [10].

Table 6.1. Modified American Joint Committee on Cancer Staging

T1		Tumor invades lamina propria or submucosa
T2		Tumor invades muscularis propria or submucosa
T3		Tumor penetrates serosa (visceral peritoneum)
T4		Tumor invades adjacent structure
N0		No regional node involved
N1		Metastasis to 1–6 regional nodes
N2		Metastasis to 7–15 regional nodes
N3		Greater than 15 nodes affected
Stage grouping	IA	T1 N0 M0
	IB	T1 N1 or T2 N0
	Stage II	T1 N2 or T2 N1
	Stage III	T1–T2 N2
		T2–T3 N1
	Stage IV	T4 N1–N3
		T3 and N3
		or metastasis

Gastroesophageal junction cancers can be staged differently, and Siewert and Stein have developed a classification system for these cancers [11]. They are divided according to the surgical approaches required for resection: type I is adenocarcinoma of the distal esophagus, which usually arises from Barrett esophagus; type II is adenocarcinoma of the stomach, which arises from the epithelium of the cardia; and type III is adenocarcinoma of the subcardial stomach. Type I adenocarcinomas often require esophagectomy, whereas types II and III can be treated by extended gastrectomy (see Chapter 5).

The postoperative systemic therapy of gastric cancer is also dictated by the type of surgery and surgical results. Patients who undergo limited perigastric lymph node dissection are considered to have had a D1 resection, while those who undergo resection that includes regional lymph nodes outside the perigastric area are considered to have undergone a D2 resection. Whether more extensive D2 resections lead to improved survival has been controversial. A randomized study from the Netherlands showed no difference in survival between D2 and D1 dissections [12], despite retrospective data from Asia suggesting otherwise [5]. A recent randomized study from Japan showed that survival of patients undergoing a D2 resection with para-aortic nodal dissection was no better than that of those treated with D2 dissection alone [13]. Patients who have undergone a complete resection with

Table 6.2. Antitumor activity of selected chemotherapy agents in advanced gastric cancer [5, 14, 15, 16]

Drug		Response rate (%)
Fluorinated pyrimidines	5-FU	
	Capecitabine	20–25
	UFT	
	S1	
Anthracyclines	Doxorubicin	17
	Epirubicin	19
Taxanes	Paclitaxel	
	Docetaxel	15–20

5-FU, 5-fluorouracil; S1, tegafur + two modulators; UFT, tegafur and uracil.

negative margins are considered to have had an R0 resection, while those with positive microscopic margins are considered to have had an R1 resection.

Systemic chemotherapy

A variety of single therapeutic chemotherapy agents and combination chemotherapy have been studied in gastric cancer. Single drugs have been given in different dosages and schedules and there have been no direct comparisons between agents. Thus, the anti-tumor activity levels, as shown in Table 6.2, are a rough estimate of efficacy.

5-Fluorouracil (5-FU), a fluorinated pyrimidine, has been the most widely studied single agent in gastric cancer. This is an antimetabolite that has been used in different schedules and dosages. Subsequently, this agent has become the standard control arm of many other single or combination chemotherapies, and experience suggests that approximately 10%–20% of patients with advanced gastric cancer (AGC) respond to this agent with an approximately 4 months' duration of response. This drug has been given by different routes and given in combination with leucovorin or folic acid. Common side-effects include mucositis, diarrhea, mild myelosuppression, and excessive tearing. Nausea is usually mild. Several oral analogs of 5-FU have been developed and studied, and three have been evaluated in gastric cancer. These include UFT (tegafur and uracil), S1 (tegafur + two modulators), and capecitabine [15, 17].

The agents UFT and S1 have undergone much more extensive testing in Japan, but given that gastric cancers occurring in Japanese people behave differently biologically to those in people from Western countries, these agents have not been adopted in the West. Capecitabine is an oral agent, and therefore is easy to administer, with an activity level comparable to that of infusional 5-FU. However, it produces mucocutaneous toxicity, which requires very careful monitoring and management [17].

In the 1980s, cisplatin was shown to have activity against gastric cancer. The major toxicities for cisplatin are nausea, vomiting, peripheral neuropathy, nephropathy, and renal tubular defects including loss of renal magnesium. The new antiemetics significantly improve the untoward effects of cisplatin. An analog of cisplatin known as carboplatin, although useful in other conditions such as lung cancer, is not that effective in gastric cancers. Oxaliplatin, another analog which has a significant antitumor activity in colon cancer, has also been tested in gastric cancers. Its activity in combination chemotherapy is discussed below [18].

More recently, taxanes such as paclitaxel and docetaxel have been studied as single agents, particularly in adenocarcinomas of the gastroesophageal junction. Docetaxel as a single agent has been shown to have activity in approximately 20% of tumors [15]. The major toxicities of this agent include alopecia, allergic reactions, edema, significant neutropenia, and effects on the nails. The average duration of response is about 6 months. This agent has now been approved for use in combination with 5-fluorouracil and cisplatin.

Anthracyclines such as doxorubicin were shown to have activity in gastric cancer in the 1970s. In Europe, an analog of anthracycline known as epirubicin has been shown to have approximately 19% activity with fewer side-effects. Anthracyclines can cause nausea, hair loss, myelosuppression, and dose-dependent cardiac toxicity [5].

The fifth class of drugs that have an antitumor effect in gastric cancers belong to the camptothecins represented by irinotecan. Camptothecins are naturally occurring alkaloids and irinotecan is cleaved in the liver to generate the active metabolite known as SN-38. The drug has modest antitumor activity, and major toxicities include myelosuppression and severe diarrhea in some patients [17, 18].

Combination chemotherapy

There is excellent evidence for combining chemotherapy agents that have different mechanisms of action and non-overlapping toxicities. Animal and clinical studies have shown that combination chemotherapy in many instances is superior to single agents. Beginning in 1990, several randomized studies have been performed to evaluate combination chemotherapy against 5-FU alone in gastric cancer. One study that combined 5-FU with cisplatin showed no significant improvement in survival over single-agent 5-FU [19]. The European Organization for Research and Treatment of Cancer (EORTC) developed a regimen consisting of a combination of 5-FU, doxorubicin, and high-dose methotrexate (FAMTX) [20]. However, this regimen failed to demonstrate any superiority over other combination regimens. Subsequently in the UK, a combination of epirubicin, cisplatin, and 5-FU (ECF) was shown to be superior to FAMTX in terms of survival. Until recently this regimen was considered the standard arm against which other combination chemotherapy regimens were evaluated [21]. These agents are highlighted in Table 6.3.

Newer generation of combination chemotherapy

Recently, a number of agents including irinotecan, S1, capecitabine, paclitaxel, and docetaxel have been intensively investigated in combination throughout the world [18]. Table 6.4 shows the results of recently conducted randomized trials with new-generation regimens.

Table 6.3. Selected combined chemotherapy regimens in advanced gastric cancer

Combination	Response rate (%)	Median survival (months)
Cisplatin + 5-FU	20–36	7–9
Epirubicin + cisplatin + 5-FU	41	9.9
Docetaxel + cisplatin + 5-FU	37	9.2

Table 6.4. Recent randomized Phase III trials in advanced gastric cancer

Regimen	No. of patients	Response	Median survival (months)	P value
FAMTX vs.	130	21	5.8	
ECF	126	46	8.9	0.0009
DCF vs.	111	39	10.2	
CF	112	21	8.5	0.0064

FAMTX, 5-FU + doxorubicin + methotrexate; DCF, docetaxel + cisplatin + 5-FU; CF, cisplatin + 5-FU.

5-FU-based regimens

With the success of FOLFOX (5-FU, leucovorin, oxaliplatin) combination chemo-therapy in colon cancer, it was natural to extend the studies of these drugs to the treatment of advanced gastric cancer. Myelosuppression, mucositis, and diarrhea are typical for this combination chemotherapy, and in a Phase II study median time to progression of disease was 5–6 months while overall survival was 10–12 months [22].

One of the studies compared a combination of docetaxel plus cisplatin and 5-FU (DCF) to cisplatin and 5-fluorouracil (CF) in 457 patients [23]. The final results showed superiority of DCF over CF in terms of disease-free as well as overall survival. Although the results were statistically significant, the improvement in survival was marginal (9.2 versus 8.6 months) [23]. Furthermore, DCF was associated with more neutropenic fever, infections, and diarrhea. These studies, however, do show that docetaxel has considerable activity in gastric cancer and should be considered as part of combination chemotherapy in future studies. The DCF was associated with significant toxicity: 81% of all patients receiving DCF had at least one great and three or four mild bouts of hematologic toxicity as well as significant mucosal toxicity, and 30% of the patients receiving DCF had neutropenic fever as compared to 13.5% of the patients receiving CF. However, the treatment-related mortality was not different in the two arms. Several variations in the dosages and schedules of DCF are being developed [24].

There are several studies in Japan which have looked at different combin-ations with S1 and UFT, but, as previously discussed, Japanese gastric patients have different biology and therefore these results may not be applicable to the US population [4].

Irinotecan-based regimens

Studies combining irinotecan with 5-FU/leucovorin showed no significant improve-ment in survival. Cisplatin is a commonly used drug in gastric cancer and thus has been combined with irinotecan. In single-arm studies, the combination therapy results were encouraging, but more studies are needed [18].

ECF-based regimens

A study known as REAL2 (randomized multi-center Phase III study, compar-ing capecitabine with 5-flourouracil and oxaliplatin with cisplatin in patients

Table 6.5. REAL-2 regimens

E	Epirubicin
C	Cisplatin
F	5-FU
E	Epirubicin
O	Oxaliplatin
F	5-FU
E	Epirubicin
C	Cisplatin
X	Capecitabine
E	Epirubicin
O	Oxaliplatin
X	Capecitabine

with advanced cancer was recently reported (Table 6.5). The study used ECF as standard treatment but used several modifications, including substituting capecitabine for 5-FU and oxaliplatin for cisplatin. This was a 2 × 2 design, and thus had four arms (ECF, EOF, ECX, EOX). In total 1002 patients were randomized and studied, and the response rates were quite similar, showing that one can substitute capecitabine for 5-FU and oxaliplatin for cisplatin in a triplet regimen [25].

Thus, in contrast to the older generation regimens, all clinical trials with newer combination chemotherapy show improved survival over single-agent chemotherapy. The DCF regimen shows a significant survival benefit, but is not accepted globally as standard treatment because of substantial toxicity. A meta-analysis performed by Wagner *et al.* [14] indicates that combination chemotherapy is better than single-agent treatment. It suggests that a regimen of three drugs including cisplatin, a fluoropyrimidine, and an anthracycline offers the most benefit.

Future prospects

Two major strategies have been used to achieve further progress in chemotherapy for gastric cancers. The first is optimization of conventional cytotoxic regimens and the second is incorporation of new active agents, particularly targeted agents for this disease. Several studies incorporating irinotecan or taxane-based therapies are currently under way all over the world.

Targeted therapy

With tremendous advances in molecular and cellular biology, a large number of molecular "targets" have been identified in various tumors. These targets can be attacked with either antibodies or small molecules.

Agents targeting the human epidermal growth factor receptor family

Four human epidermal growth factor receptors have been identified. This family is made up of tyrosine kinase growth factor receptors which regulate signal transduction in cellular processes including proliferation, differentiation, and apoptosis [26].

The epidermal growth factor receptor (EGFR) is a 170-kDa transmembrane protein with intrinsic tyrosine kinase activity, and has at least four family members: EGFR, erbb-2 (also designated as neu and HER), erbb-3, and erbb-4. These families regulate cell growth, proliferation, and differentiation, primarily of tissues of epithelial origin. When EGF family members bind to receptors of the EGFR family, the tyrosine kinase domain of the receptor undergoes phosphorylation and triggers a cascade of downstream biochemical reactions, resulting in signal transduction. The EGFR signaling system is tightly regulated in normal tissue, and is overexpressed, mutated, or overproduced in neoplastic disease. A number of agents which bind to and inhibit EGFR have been tested in tumors and others are being evaluated [26].

Gefitinib, a small-molecule inhibitor of tyrosine kinase, blocks EGFR and was first investigated for single-agent therapy of gastric cancer. The studies showed this agent to have very modest activity. A Phase II study with erlotinib, another EGFR tyrosine kinase inhibitor, showed a response rate of 9% [27]. This led investigators to widen the studies of EGFR inhibitors such as trastuzumab (Herceptin), an antibody against HER-2/neu. In a large ongoing Phase III study of 2691 patients, the patients were randomized to either cisplatin and a pyrimidine analog or the same agents plus Herceptin. Of these 2691 patients, 584 (21.7%) were found to be positive for HER-2/neu. However, when different subtypes of cancer were considered, gastroesophageal junction cancer had a 34.8% HER-2 positivity as judged by immunohistochemistry, while only 19.8% of stomach cancers were HER-2/neu positive. In patients with intestinal-type tumors, 31.8% had HER-2/neu positivity compared with only 6.2% of patients with diffuse histology [28]. These studies further illustrate that gastroesophageal junction adenocarcinomas have a different biological behavior and thus may be more likely to respond to targeted therapies.

Recently, a Phase II study with cetuximab (an antibody against EGFR) in combination with 5-FU/leucovorin plus irinotecan (FOLFIRI) reported a promising response rate of 42% with a median time to progression of 8 months. Cetuximab is now often combined with other agents, leading to a high response, and this needs verification in randomized trials [29, 30]. Table 6.6 summarizes some of these studies.

Lapatinib is a dual inhibitor of tyrosine kinase domains 1 and 2 of HER-2/neu, and interferes with autophosphorylation. Lapatinib has been shown to be active against HER-2/neu-positive breast cancer when combined with hormonal therapy as well as in combination with capecitabine. A Phase I study of lapatinib and weekly paclitaxel in gastric cancer is under way, and other studies are being proposed.

Agents targeted to vascular endothelial growth factor (VEGF)

One of the first targeted compounds studied was bevacizumab, a humanized monoclonal antibody that binds to the vascular endothelial growth factor (VEGF) ligand. This is expressed in most solid tumors and tumor stromal cells [31]. VEGF inhibitors have been shown to have significant activity in colorectal cancer in combination with chemotherapy. A Phase II trial of bevacizumab combined with irinotecan and cisplatin had a response rate of 65% [32]. Bevacizumab can cause serious side-effects including cardiac and cerebral ischemic episodes in brain and heart tissue, as well as gastric perforations. Venous thromboembolism is also a known complication [33]. There is an ongoing randomized trial comparing capecitabine plus

Table 6.6. Results of "targeted" therapy in advanced gastric cancer outcomes

Agent		Outcomes (%)
I. EGFR inhibitor	Gefitinib	SD 18
	Erlotinib[a]	CR 1
	Matuzumab	PR 8
		SD 39
II. Anti-angiogenesis	Bevacizumab	SD 38
	Sunitinib	PR 5
		SD 36

[a] All GE junction adenocarcinomas.

CR, complete response; PR, partial response; SD, stabilization of disease. Trastuzumab (Herceptin) is currently being evaluated.

cisplatin with these two agents combined with bevacizumab as first-line therapy. More recently, small-molecule inhibitors of the VEGF receptor tyrosine kinase have been developed. Sunitinib, which has significant antitumor activity in renal cell carcinoma, was shown to have modest activity against gastric tumors [34].

Other targeted agents

Other agents including inhibitors of mTOR (mammalian target of rapamycin) are currently being studied for their efficacy in gastric cancer [35]. The C-MET proto-oncogene encodes a transmembrane tyrosine kinase receptor (hepatocyte growth factor), which may play a role in gastric cancer. A high level of MET expression has been correlated with recurrence and poor survival in several tumors including those in lung and gastric tissue [36]; agents that target elevated C-MET are undergoing evaluation at this time [37]. Lastly, the NF-kappa-B family of inducible transcription factors is involved in tumor promotion, angiogenesis, and metastasis, as well as inflammation. Because of its diverse effects, inhibiting NF-kappa-B is a double-edged sword, but it can be targeted through proteasome inhibitors such as bortezomib. A Phase II trial with this agent showed a modest effect in gastric cancer [17, 38].

Role of chemotherapy in metastatic disease

In advanced and metastatic gastric carcinoma, single-agent or combination chemotherapy clearly has modest activity. Therefore, it has been appropriate to ask whether it is worthwhile using palliative chemotherapy rather than the best available supportive treatments. Wagner *et al.* performed a meta-analysis [14] of trials that looked at best supportive care versus systemic chemotherapy. The authors conclude that median and overall survival are better in patients receiving chemotherapy as compared to those receiving best supportive care, with a hazard ratio of 0.39 in favor of chemotherapy. Median survival was increased from 4.3 months for best supportive care to approximately 11 months for chemotherapy. In these studies, the quality of life was not formally assessed, and therefore it is difficult to evaluate whether improved survival was associated with improved quality of life. However, based on the results of this study, it is appropriate to consider palliative chemotherapy in AGC.

Role of chemotherapy in localized disease

Currently, the reported 5-year survival rates with resected Stage II, IIIa, IIIb, and IV gastric cancers are 34%, 20%, 8%, and 7% respectively. Further, intra-abdominal recurrence rate after surgery alone is 70% [39]. These poor results suggest that surgery alone for locally advanced disease is not sufficient and that other approaches must be taken to reduce the risk of recurrence.

Neoadjuvant chemotherapy

Neoadjuvant chemotherapy is associated with several advantages including enhanced delivery of drug in the preoperative setting due to intact vasculature, as well as potential down-staging of the tumor before surgery, allowing a more complete resection of neoplastic tissue. Neoadjuvant chemotherapy also allows identification of patients who are likely to develop early metastasis, thereby avoiding the morbidity of a major surgical procedure. The drawbacks of neoadjuvant chemotherapy include delayed surgery and a probable increase in postsurgical morbidity and mortality. The UK National Cancer Research Institute Upper GI Clinical Studies Group (called MAGIC) conducted a Phase III clinical trial (Table 6.7) to determine whether preoperative chemotherapy can be translated into a survival advantage in patients with operable disease [40]. Between 1994 and 2002, 503 patients with adenocarcinoma of the stomach (74%), the esophagogastric junction (15%) or lower esophagus (11%) were deemed suitable for resection and were randomized to receive preoperative radiochemotherapy (250 patients for surgery alone, 253 who received combined surgery and preoperative chemotherapy). The chemotherapy consisted of 21-day cycles of epirubicin (50 mg/m^2), cisplatin (60 mg/m^2), and continuous infusion of 5-FU (200 mg/m^2 daily) (ECF) given in three preoperative and three postoperative cycles.

The vast majority of the patients (88%) completed preoperative chemotherapy, while only 55% who were started on postoperative therapy were able to finish. In all, 40% of patients completed all six cycles of chemotherapy. Results from the 500 patients showed that preoperative chemotherapy had a significant benefit, particularly in those patients with locally advanced disease. The hazard ratio was 0.7 (95% confidence interval of 0.56–0.80; $p = 0.002$) for disease-free survival and was 0.80 (95% confidence interval of 0.6–1.08; $p = 0.06$) for overall survival in favor of the chemotherapy arm. The postoperative complications were similar in both.

Table 6.7. Chemotherapy schedule for MAGIC

ECF × 3 cycles	→	SURGERY	→	ECF × 3 cycles

C, cisplatin; E, epirubicin; F, 5-fluorouracil.

Furthermore, patients receiving preoperative chemotherapy had significantly more down-staging of their disease and had an increased rate of curative resection. A recent update has shown a definite benefit with a median survival of 24 months compared to 20 months with surgery alone (hazard ratio is 0.75; 95% confidence interval is 0.60–0.9; $p = 0.009$) [41].

Another approach used has been to give preoperative chemotherapy followed by postoperative intraperitoneal (IP) chemotherapy to prevent the local relapse so commonly seen in gastric cancers. Crookes *et al.* conducted a study of 59 patients with resectable gastric adenocarcinoma and administered two cycles of preoperative infusional 5-FU together with leucovorin and cisplatin. This was followed by surgery and two additional cycles of intraperitoneal 5-FU and cisplatin 3–4 weeks postoperatively. A high proportion of these patients went on to have surgery (95%) with 70% of the patients undergoing surgery with curative intent. The median follow-up was 45 months, at which point only 23% of the patients who had undergone a curative resection had relapsed [42].

More recently, Newman *et al.* conducted a similar study with two cycles of irinotecan and cisplatin followed by surgery and IP chemotherapy with floxuridine and cisplatin. Of the 32 evaluable patients, 29 (90.6%) underwent surgery. Of the 25 patients who underwent surgery with curative intent, there were no local recurrences [43]. These studies need confirmation with Phase III randomized trials.

Yan *et al.* recently conducted a systematic meta-analysis of trials with adjuvant intraperitoneal chemotherapy in gastric cancer. The authors extracted 13 randomized controlled trials, of which 10 were judged to be of fair quality for analysis. The data suggest that there was significant improvement in survival with hyperthermic intraoperative IP chemotherapy, or with this therapy along with early postoperative IP chemotherapy (hazard ratio = 0.45; 95% CI = 0.29–0.6; $p = 0.000\ 2$). This survival improvement was not seen with normothermic intraoperative IP treatment [44]. The majority of these trials were performed in Japan, and it is difficult to know whether the results can be extrapolated to Western countries. Further, most of these trials had major deficiencies and there is a need for a prospective large randomized trial to address this issue [44].

Preoperative radiation

In tumors of the gastric body, a role for neoadjuvant radiation is supported by a randomized trial from China of 370 patients, which showed an 18% increase in the rate of radical resection with neoadjuvant radiotherapy to 40 Gy in 20 fractions. Patients who received preoperative radiation had a significantly increased over-all survival at 10 years (20% vs. 13%, p = 0.009) [45]. These improvements were achieved without an increase in treatment-related morbidity or operative mortality. Three trials from Russia have also suggested a survival benefit of preoperative radiation [46].

Preoperative chemoradiation

The role of neoadjuvant chemoradiation in patients with gastric cancer has been the subject of interest due to the success of this approach in other GI malignancies. The growing role of neoadjuvant chemoradiation of carcinomas of the gastroesophageal junction stems from the success of this approach in the setting of esophageal cancer [47]. The CALGB study 9781, which accrued only 56 patients, showed a survival benefit for neoadjuvant chemoradiation with cisplatin/5-FU in combination with radiotherapy [48]. Adenocarcinomas made up 75% of the tumors, most of which were located at the gastroesophageal junction.

The MD Anderson Cancer Center pioneered an approach using induction chemotherapy followed by chemoradiation and surgery for tumors of the gastric body. This was validated in the cooperative group setting with a Phase II trial, RTOG 9904. Induction chemotherapy was with 5-FU (200 mg/m^2 per day, infusion on days 1–21) and with cisplatin (20 mg/m^2 per day on days 1–5) for two cycles, followed by radiotherapy to 45 Gy in 25 fractions, with concurrent 5-FU (300 mg/m^2) and paclitaxel (45 mg/m^2) each Monday. Chemoradiation was followed by a D2 surgical resection. With 43 patients available for analysis, the pathologic complete remission rate was 26%, and the rate of R0 resection was 77%. The median survival was 23.2 months, and 72% of patients were alive at 1 year. At 1 year, 82% of those with a complete remission were alive versus 69% of those with less than a complete remission. However, 21% of patients developed grade 4 toxicity, making this a difficult regimen to tolerate [49].

Postoperative chemotherapy

The goal of systemic chemotherapy in the postoperative setting is to target residual micrometastasis after surgical resection in an attempt to increase disease-free and overall survival. As a significant number of patients with gastric cancer develop local recurrence, the use of chemotherapy alone with the systemic treatment has been disappointing. A large number of studies conducted in Japan and in Western countries over several decades have failed to demonstrate a survival advantage with adjuvant chemotherapy alone. Although some studies with agents such as mitomycin-C conducted in Japan indicated a benefit in terms of survival, these results have not been consistently reproduced. The combination of 5-FU, doxorubicin, and mitomycin-C (FAM) was compared with surgery alone by Coombes *et al.* and no difference in disease-free or overall survival was found [50]. Other investigators have confirmed these negative results. Italian investigators used a combination of etoposide, doxorubicin, and cisplatin in a randomized trial, but observed no improvement in survival over surgery alone [51].

A large number of studies and meta-analyses have been conducted addressing the efficacy of adjuvant chemotherapy. Most of these meta-analyses show a small survival benefit with adjuvant chemotherapy as compared to surgery alone (odds ratio = 0.80; 95% CI = 0.66–0.97) [16]. Based on this analysis, most authors recommend routine use of adjuvant chemotherapy in patients with gastric cancer following resection. However, it should be noted that chemotherapy regimens used in many of these adjuvant trials were suboptimal and therefore these unimpressive results are not unexpected [52].

Postoperative combination of radiation and chemotherapy

The Mayo Clinic began a series of studies in the 1960s using postoperative radiation and 5-FU chemotherapy as adjuvant therapy in a number of gastrointestinal malignancies including gastric cancer. These studies indicated a rather significant improvement in survival with a combination of 5-FU and radiation therapy compared with surgery alone [53, 54]. These trials were criticized because a high proportion of patients did not receive the assigned therapy.

The landmark GI Intergroup 0116 trial demonstrated a survival benefit of adjuvant chemoradiation. In the trial, 556 patients who underwent complete resection of a locally advanced (T2–4 or N+) gastric or gastroesophageal junction adenocarcinoma (20%) were randomized to surgery alone or combined modality therapy. The chemoradiation arm received one cycle of 5-FU/leucovorin (425 mg/m^2 days 1–5), followed by chemoradiation to 45 Gy in 25 fractions with bolus 5-FU/leucovorin (400 mg/m^2 per day) the first 4 and last 3 days of radiation. They then received two 5-day cycles of adjuvant 5-FU/leucovorin. With a median follow-up of 5 years, the median survival was 36 months in the chemoradiation therapy group and 27 months in the surgery-alone group. The hazard ratio for death was 1.35 (95% CI = 1.09–1.66, $p = 0.005$) for the surgery-alone arm. Local recurrence occurred in 29% of surgical patients and 19% of those in the chemoradiation therapy group. The rate of regional relapse (peritoneal carcinomatosis) was reduced from 72% to 65% [39]. This study has been criticized due to the minimal extent of surgery (54% had D0 dissection), suggesting that radiotherapy may have compensated for inadequate surgical resection. However, a non-randomized study in South Korea, where all patients underwent a D2 dissection, showed a similar benefit to those who received chemoradiation versus those who did not [55]. Thus, it is controversial whether perioperative chemotherapy or postoperative chemoradiation is the true standard of care [5, 10, 56, 57].

Comprehensive care for the patient with gastric cancer

Comprehensive care for the patient with gastric cancer includes treatment for complications that occur as a result of surgery, radiation, and chemotherapy. Patients with gastric cancer who have undergone gastrectomy often develop a dumping syndrome characterized by diarrhea and cramping as well as palpitations. Patients also develop malabsorption of B12, iron, and calcium that needs to be treated. Radiation can cause diarrhea and nausea in the short term and has associated risks of bowel obstruction or kidney damage in the long term. The potential late effects of chemotherapy depend on the drugs used. For example, cisplatin may cause peripheral neuropathy, while anthracyclines may cause dose-dependent cardiomyopathy. These need to be monitored subsequent to the patient's treatment [5, 8].

Immunochemotherapy

Investigators have evaluated giving immunostimulants along with cytotoxic chemotherapy and radiation therapy. Most of these trials have been small and are difficult to interpret. The most studied compound is the protein-bound polysaccharide of a *Streptococcus pyogenes* preparation known as OK432. Studies using this agent have produced variable results but suggest a possible antitumor effect [58]. Larger studies are needed to evaluate this approach.

Recommendations

In summary, the management of the patient with gastric cancer remains challenging as results continue to be unsatisfactory. Patients presenting with resected gastric or gastroesophageal junction carcinoma should be evaluated and treated in a multidisciplinary setting. If a clinical trial is available, it should be offered to the patient. If the patient is not part of a clinical trial, he or she should be offered preoperative chemotherapy, which includes three cycles of induction chemotherapy followed by surgery and then an additional three cycles of chemotherapy. This should be discussed along with the data for adjuvant chemoradiation, and the relative risks and benefits of each approach.

Many patients, however, are referred to medical oncology after they have undergone gastric resection. Whether their survival is enhanced by D1 or D2 lymph node dissection remains controversial. There is no question that those patients who have no residual disease (R0) do better than those whose disease is left behind (R1). In the absence of a clinical trial, these patients should be treated based on the results of Intergroup Study 0116 with chemotherapy followed by radiation and then additional chemotherapy as shown in Table 6.8. Whether ECF or DCF should replace 5-FU/leucovorin for the first two and the last two cycles of chemotherapy is open to question.

Patients with a good performance status who present with metastatic gastric cancer should be offered chemotherapy. The choice between a DCF- or ECF-based regimen depends on the performance status of the patient, as DCF is a much more toxic therapy. In order to enhance the effectiveness of the current therapy, clinical trials are essential and several are based on new targeted therapies such as EGFR blockers. In this context, the new finding that approximately one-third of patients with gastroesophageal junction adenocarcinoma are positive for HER-2/neu suggests the possibility of using Herceptin in this disease. Thus, there is a need for a more aggressive approach with new therapy in gastric cancer.

The early diagnosis of gastric and gastroesophageal junction tumors remains a challenge. The application of new imaging modalities such as endoscopic

Table 6.8. Gastric adjuvant therapy Intergroup Trial 0116

Resected	5-FU + LV		Radiation +		5-FU + LV
Ib – IV M0	→	Two cycles	→	5-FU + LV	→	Two cycles

5-FU, 5-fluorouracil; LV, leucovorin.

ultrasonography and molecular imaging with MRI may facilitate early detection. Patients with gastric cancer associated with *H. pylori* should be treated for the bacterium, but it is unclear whether this will affect recurrence or the development of a new primary within any residual stomach tissue.

It now appears that many, if not all, cancers originate from cancer stem cells. In a mouse model there is evidence that *H. pylori*-induced gastric cancer may originate from bone-marrow-derived stem cells. If confirmed, this will open new avenues of therapy [59]. Clearly, given the poor outcomes associated with treatment of locally advanced gastric carcinoma, early detection, new therapeutic strategies, and novel therapeutic approaches are sorely needed.

REFERENCES

1. Jemal A, Siegel R, Ward E *et al.* Cancer statistics, 2008. *CA Cancer J Clin* 2008; **58**(2): 71–96.
2. Correa P. Human gastric carcinogenesis: a multistep and multifactorial process – first American Cancer Society Award Lecture on Cancer Epidemiology and Prevention. *Cancer Res* 1992; **52**(24): 6735–40.
3. McNamara D and El-Omar E. *Helicobacter pylori* infection and the pathogenesis of gastric cancer: a paradigm for host-bacterial interactions. *Dig Liver Dis* 2008; **40**(7): 504–9.
4. Ohtsu A, Yoshida S, and Saijo N. Disparities in gastric cancer chemotherapy between the East and West. *J Clin Oncol* 2006; **24**(14): 2188–96.
5. Pisters WT, Kelsen DP, and Tepper JE. Cancer of the stomach. In Devita VT Jr., Helman S, Rosenberg S eds., *Cancer: Principles and Practices of Oncology*. Philadelphia, PA: Lippincott, Williams and Wilkins, 2008; pp. 1043–78.
6. Brenner B, Tang LH, Shia J, Klimstra DS, and Kelsen DP. Small cell carcinomas of the gastrointestinal tract: clinicopathological features and treatment approach. *Semin Oncol* 2007; **34**(1): 43–50.
7. Islami F and Kamangar F. *Helicobacter pylori* and esophageal cancer risk: a meta-analysis. *Cancer Prev Res* 2008; **1**(5): 329–38.
8. Minsky BD. Chemotherapy and radiation therapy for gastric cancer. In Rustgi AK ed., *Gastrointestinal Cancer*. Edinburgh: WB Saunders, 2002; pp. 344–50.
9. Kwee RM and Kwee TC. Imaging in local staging of gastric cancer: a systematic review. *J Clin Oncol* 2007; **25**(15): 2107–16.
10. Moehler M, Galle PR, Gockel I, Junginger T, and Schmidberger H. The multidisciplinary management of gastrointestinal cancer. Multimodal treatment of gastric cancer. *Best Pract Res Clin Gastroenterol* 2007; **21**(6): 965–81.
11. Siewert JR and Stein HJ. Classification of adenocarcinoma of the oesophagogastric junction. *Br J Surg* 1998; **85**(11): 1457–9.

12. Bonenkamp JJ, Hermans J, Sasako M *et al.* Extended lymph-node dissection for gastric cancer. *N Engl J Med* 1999; **340**(12): 908–14.

13. Sasako M, Sano T, Yamamoto S *et al.* D2 lymphadenectomy alone or with para-aortic nodal dissection for gastric cancer. *N Engl J Med* 2008; **359**(5): 453–62.

14. Wagner AD, Grothe W, Behl S *et al.* Chemotherapy for advanced gastric cancer. *Cochrane Database Syst Rev* 2005(2): CD004064.

15. Wagner AD, Grothe W, Haerting J, Kleber G, Grothey A, and Fleig WE. Chemotherapy in advanced gastric cancer: a systematic review and meta-analysis based on aggregate data. *J Clin Oncol* 2006; **24**(18): 2903–9.

16. Wagner AD, Schneider PM, and Fleig WE. The role of chemotherapy in patients with established gastric cancer. *Best Pract Res Clin Gastroenterol* 2006; **20**(4): 789–99.

17. Ohtsu A. Chemotherapy for metastatic gastric cancer: past, present, and future. *J Gastroenterol* 2008; **43**(4): 256–64.

18. Lordick F and Jager D. Current status and future of chemotherapy and biochemotherapy in esophageal cancers. *Gastrointest Cancer Res* 2008; **2**(4): 187–97.

19. Kim NK, Park YS, Heo DS *et al.* A phase III randomized study of 5-fluorouracil and cisplatin versus 5-fluorouracil, doxorubicin, and mitomycin C versus 5-fluorouracil alone in the treatment of advanced gastric cancer. *Cancer* 1993; **71**(12): 3813–18.

20. Wils JA, Klein HO, Wagener DJ *et al.* Sequential high-dose methotrexate and fluorouracil combined with doxorubicin – a step ahead in the treatment of advanced gastric cancer: a trial of the European Organization for Research and Treatment of Cancer Gastrointestinal Tract Cooperative Group. *J Clin Oncol* 1991; **9**(5): 827–31.

21. Webb A, Cunningham D, Scarffe JH *et al.* Randomized trial comparing epirubicin, cisplatin, and fluorouracil versus fluorouracil, doxorubicin, and methotrexate in advanced esophagogastric cancer. *J Clin Oncol* 1997; **15**(1): 261–7.

22. Keam B, Im SA, Han SW *et al.* Modified FOLFOX-6 chemotherapy in advanced gastric cancer: Results of phase II study and comprehensive analysis of polymorphisms as a predictive and prognostic marker. *BMC Cancer* 2008; **8**: 148.

23. Van Cutsem E, Moiseyenko VM, Tjulandin S *et al.* Phase III study of docetaxel and cisplatin plus fluorouracil compared with cisplatin and fluorouracil as first-line therapy for advanced gastric cancer: a report of the V325 Study Group. *J Clin Oncol* 2006; **24**(31): 4991–7.

24. Ajani JA. Optimizing docetaxel chemotherapy in patients with cancer of the gastric and gastroesophageal junction: evolution of the docetaxel, cisplatin, and 5-fluorouracil regimen. *Cancer* 2008; **113**(5): 945–55.

25. Cunningham D, Starling N, Rao S *et al.* Capecitabine and oxaliplatin for advanced esophagogastric cancer. *N Engl J Med* 2008; **358**(1): 36–46.

26. Karamouzis MV, Grandis JR, and Argiris A. Therapies directed against epidermal growth factor receptor in aerodigestive carcinomas. *J Am Med Assoc* 2007; **298**(1): 70–82.

27. Dragovich T, McCoy S, Fenoglio-Preiser CM *et al.* Phase II trial of erlotinib in gastroe-sophageal junction and gastric adenocarcinomas: SWOG 0127. *J Clin Oncol* 2006; **24**(30): 4922–7.

28. Bang Y, Chung H, Sawaki A *et al.* HER2-positivity rates in advanced gastric cancer (GC): results from a large international phase III trial. *J Clin Oncol* (Meeting Abstracts) 2008; **26**(15 Suppl): 4526.

29. Milas L, Raju U, Liao Z, and Ajani J. Targeting molecular determinants of tumor chemo-radioresistance. *Semin Oncol* 2005; **32**(6 Suppl 9): S78–S81.

30. Pinto C, Di Fabio F, Siena S *et al.* Phase II study of cetuximab in combination with FOLFIRI in patients with untreated advanced gastric or gastroesophageal junction adenocarcinoma (FOLCETUX study). *Ann Oncol* 2007; **18**(3): 510–17.

31. Lieto E, Ferraraccio F, Orditura M *et al.* Expression of vascular endothelial growth factor (VEGF) and epidermal growth factor receptor (EGFR) is an independent prognostic indicator of worse outcome in gastric cancer patients. *Ann Surg Oncol* 2008; **15**(1): 69–79.

32. Shah MA, Ramanathan RK, Ilson DH *et al.* Multicenter phase II study of irinotecan, cisplatin, and bevacizumab in patients with metastatic gastric or gastroesophageal junction adenocarcin-oma. *J Clin Oncol* 2006; **24**(33): 5201–6.

33. Elice F, Jacoub J, Rickles FR, Falanga A, and Rodeghiero F. Hemostatic complications of angio-genesis inhibitors in cancer patients. *Am J Hematol* 2008; **83**(11): 862–70.

34. Bang Y, Kang Y, Kang W *et al.* Sunitinib as second-line treatment for advanced gastric cancer: preliminary results from a phase II study. *J Clin Oncol* (Meeting Abstracts) 2007; **25**(18 suppl): 4603.

35. Lang SA, Gaumann A, Koehl GE *et al.* Mammalian target of rapamycin is activated in human gastric cancer and serves as a target for therapy in an experimental model. *Int J Cancer* 2007; **120**(8): 1803–10.

36. Nakajima M, Sawada H, Yamada Y *et al.* The prognostic significance of amplification and overexpression of c-met and c-erb B-2 in human gastric carcinomas. *Cancer* 1999; **85**(9): 1894–902.

37. Christensen JG, Schreck R, Burrows J *et al.* A selective small molecule inhibitor of c-Met kinase inhibits c-Met-dependent phenotypes in vitro and exhibits cytoreductive antitumor activity in vivo. *Cancer Res* 2003; **63**(21): 7345–55.

38. Cervantes A, Rosello S, Roda D, and Rodriguez-Braun E. The treatment of advanced gastric cancer: current strategies and future perspectives. *Ann Oncol* 2008; **19**(Suppl 5): v103–7.

39. Macdonald JS, Smalley SR, Benedetti J *et al.* Chemoradiotherapy after surgery compared with surgery alone for adenocarcinoma of the stomach or gastroesophageal junction. *N Engl J Med* 2001; **345**(10): 725–30.

40. Cunningham D, Allum WH, Stenning SP *et al.* Perioperative chemotherapy versus surgery alone for resectable gastroesophageal cancer. *N Engl J Med* 2006; **355**(1): 11–20.

41. Cunningham D, Allum WH, Stenning SP, Weeden S, for the NUGICCSG. Perioperative chemotherapy in operable gastric and lower oesophageal cancer: final results of a randomised, controlled trial (the MAGIC trial, ISRCTN 93793971). *J Clin Oncol* (Meeting Abstracts) 2005; **23**(16 Suppl): 4001.

42. Crookes P, Leichman CG, Leichman L *et al.* Systemic chemotherapy for gastric carcinoma followed by postoperative intraperitoneal therapy: a final report. *Cancer* 1997; **79**(9): 1767–75.

43. Newman E, Potmesil M, Ryan T *et al.* Neoadjuvant chemotherapy, surgery, and adjuvant intraperitoneal chemotherapy in patients with locally advanced gastric or gastroesophageal junction carcinoma: a phase II study. *Semin Oncol* 2005; **32**(6 Suppl 9): S97–S100.

44. Yan TD, Black D, Sugarbaker PH *et al.* A systematic review and meta-analysis of the randomized controlled trials on adjuvant intraperitoneal chemotherapy for resectable gastric cancer. *Ann Surg Oncol* 2007; **14**(10): 2702–13.

45. Zhang ZX, Gu XZ, Yin WB, Huang GJ, Zhang DW, and Zhang RG. Randomized clinical trial on the combination of preoperative irradiation and surgery in the treatment of adenocarcinoma of gastric cardia (AGC) – report on 370 patients. *Int J Radiat Oncol Biol Phys* 1998; **42**(5): 929–34.

46. Shchepotin IB, Evans SR, Chorny V *et al.* Intensive preoperative radiotherapy with local hyperthermia for the treatment of gastric carcinoma. *Surg Oncol* 1994; **3**(1): 37–44.

47. Walsh TN, Noonan N, Hollywood D, Kelly A, Keeling N, and Hennessy TP. A comparison of multimodal therapy and surgery for esophageal adenocarcinoma. *N Engl J Med* 1996; **335**(7): 462–7.

48. Tepper J, Krasna MJ, Niedzwiecki D *et al.* Phase III trial of trimodality therapy with cisplatin, fluorouracil, radiotherapy, and surgery compared with surgery alone for esophageal cancer: CALGB 9781. *J Clin Oncol* 2008; **26**(7): 1086–92.

49. Ajani JA, Winter K, Okawara GS *et al.* Phase II trial of preoperative chemoradiation in patients with localized gastric adenocarcinoma (RTOG 9904): quality of combined modality therapy and pathologic response. *J Clin Oncol* 2006; **24**(24): 3953–8.

50. Coombes RC, Schein PS, Chilvers CE *et al.* A randomized trial comparing adjuvant fluorouracil, doxorubicin, and mitomycin with no treatment in operable gastric cancer. International Collaborative Cancer Group. *J Clin Oncol* 1990; **8**(8): 1362–9.

51. Bajetta E, Buzzoni R, Mariani L *et al.* Adjuvant chemotherapy in gastric cancer: 5-year results of a randomised study by the Italian Trials in Medical Oncology (ITMO) Group. *Ann Oncol* 2002; **13**(2): 299–307.

52. Lim L, Michael M, Mann GB, and Leong T. Adjuvant therapy in gastric cancer. *J Clin Oncol* 2005; **23**(25): 6220–32.

53. Childs DS, Jr., Moertel CG, Holbrook MA, Reitemeier RJ, and Colby M, Jr. Treatment of unresectable adenocarcinomas of the stomach with a combination of 5-fluorouracil and radiation. *Am J Roentgenol Radium Ther Nucl Med* 1968; **102**(3): 541–4.

54. Moertel CG, Childs DS, O'Fallon JR, Holbrook MA, Schutt AJ, and Reitemeier RJ. Combined 5-fluorouracil and radiation therapy as a surgical adjuvant for poor prognosis gastric carcinoma. *J Clin Oncol* 1984; **2**(11): 1249–54.

55. Kim S, Lim DH, Lee J *et al.* An observational study suggesting clinical benefit for adjuvant postoperative chemoradiation in a population of over 500 cases after gastric resection with D2 nodal dissection for adenocarcinoma of the stomach. *Int J Radiat Oncol Biol Phys* 2005; **63**(5): 1279–85.

56. Coburn NG, Govindarajan A, Law CH *et al.* Stage-specific effect of adjuvant therapy following gastric cancer resection: a population-based analysis of 4,041 patients. *Ann Surg Oncol* 2008; **15**(2): 500–7.

57. Macdonald JS. Gastric cancer – new therapeutic options. *N Engl J Med* 2006; **355**(1): 76–7.

58. Sakamoto J, Teramukai S, Nakazato H *et al.* Efficacy of adjuvant immunochemotherapy with OK-432 for patients with curatively resected gastric cancer: a meta-analysis of centrally randomized controlled clinical trials. *J Immunother* 2002; **25**(5): 405–12.

59. Takaishi S, Okumura T, and Wang TC. Gastric cancer stem cells. *J Clin Oncol* 2008; **26**(17): 2876–82.

7

MDCT, EUS, PET/CT, and MRI in the management of patients with gastric neoplasms

Richard M. Gore, Jung Hoon Kim, and Chiao-Yun Chen

Adenocarcinoma of the stomach

Introduction

Since the late 1990s, the treatment of gastric cancer has become increasingly sophisticated with therapeutic options ranging from endoscopic mucosal resection (EMR) and endoscopic submucosal dissection (ESD) for selected mucosal (see Chapter 3) early gastric cancer (EGC) to more radical gastrectomy and lymph node dissection (see Chapter 5) for advanced gastric cancer (AGC). Accordingly, accurate pre-operative staging, particularly with respect to the depth of mural invasion, adjacent organ invasion, and nodal involvement, is key to selecting the most suitable therapy and avoiding inappropriate attempts at curative surgery [1, 2, 3, 4, 5, 6, 7, 8].

Although upper gastrointestinal (GI) endoscopy and double-contrast upper GI series are the primary means of diagnosing gastric cancer and are excellent in depicting the precise location of the tumor, they cannot determine the depth of mural invasion or the presence of local, regional, or distant metastases. Recent advances in multidetector computed tomography (MDCT), endoscopic ultrasound (EUS), magnetic resonance (MR) imaging, and positron emission tomography-computed tomography (PET-CT) have dramatically improved the accuracy of preoperative staging of patients with gastric cancer and have provided a more accurate means of assessing tumor response to therapy and detecting recurrent disease [9, 10, 11, 12, 13, 14, 15, 16, 17, 18].

Staging classifications

Early gastric cancer is defined as tumor limited to the mucosa and submucosa, irrespective of lymph node involvement (Figure 7.1). Although the term EGC suggests

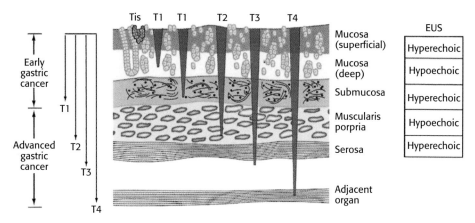

Figure 7.1. Classification of gastric adenocarcinoma by depth of invasion, the T classification. In the TNM classification, T denotes the depth of invasion of the neoplasm. Tis indicates carcinoma in situ. T1 tumors are limited to the mucosa and submucosa. This is also the depth of invasion for early gastric cancers. T2 tumors penetrate the muscularis propria but not the serosa. T3 cancers penetrate the serosa without involving adjacent organs. T4 tumors penetrate the serosa and involve adjacent organs and tissues. T2, T3, and T4 tumors are considered advanced gastric cancers. The term early gastric cancer does not consider lymph node status but merely depth of invasion. EUS: the corresponding sonographic features of the gastric wall as shown on endoscopic ultrasound. From Houghton JM and Wang TC. Tumors of the stomach. In Feldman M, Friedman LS and Brandt LJ eds., *Gastrointestinal and Liver Disease*, 8th edn. Philadelphia, PA: WB Saunders, 2005; p. 1152, Figure 52–5.

an early lesion that is confined and asymptomatic, these lesions may be large, symptomatic, and have lymph node involvement [9, 10, 11, 12]. The Japanese Research Society for Gastric Cancer has divided EGC lesions into main types and three main subtypes (Figure 7.2). Any gastric cancer that has invaded the muscularis propria is classified as an AGC. Bormann described four morphologic types of advanced gastric cancer (Figure 7.3) [19, 20, 21, 22, 23, 24].

The TNM classification scheme (Table 7.1) defined by the American Joint Committee on Cancer (AJCC) is used worldwide to provide prognostic information about gastric tumors. It classifies gastric carcinomas according to the extent of the primary tumor (T), the presence or absence of nodal metastases (N), and the presence or absence of distal metastases (M). Gastric cancers are classified into four degrees of T, four degrees of N, and two degrees of M, providing 19 categories that are then condensed down to four pathologic stages. The accuracy of pathologic staging is proportional to the number of lymph nodes examined [25, 26, 27, 28, 29].

Accurate T staging is the most significant element in selecting the appropriate therapeutic approach for the patient. T1 denotes a tumor confined to the mucosa

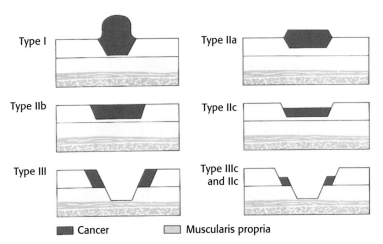

Figure 7.2. Japanese Research Society for Gastric Cancer classification of early gastric cancer. Type I = elevated lesions that protrude more than 5 mm into the lumen, usually larger than 2 cm. Type II = superficial lesions with elevated (IIa), flat (IIb), or depressed (IIc) components. Type III = excavated lesion resembling a gastric ulcer but with irregular ulcer craters, clubbing, fusion or amputation, or radiating folds and nodularity of the adjacent mucosa. Sometimes the types are combined (e.g., Type III and IIc).

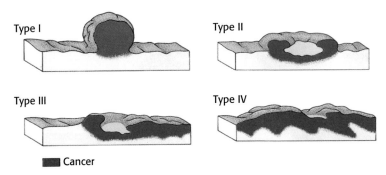

Figure 7.3. Bormann classification of advanced gastric cancer. Type I = fungating type; Type II = carcinomatous ulcer without infiltration of the surrounding mucosa; Type III = carcinomatous ulcer with infiltration of the surrounding mucosa; Type IV = a diffuse infiltrating carcinoma (linitis plastica).

and submucosa; T2 indicates tumor invading the muscularis propria; T3 denotes invasion into the serosa; and T4 indicates invasion of adjacent organs or structures [22, 23, 24].

The Japanese Research Society has the following classification system for N disease (Figure 7.4), which indicates the degree of lymph node invasion. N0 indicates no lymph node involvement; N1 denotes involvement of perigastric lymph nodes within 3 cm of the primary cancer; N2 disease indicates regional lymph node involvement (left gastric, common hepatic, splenic, and celiac) more than

Table 7.1. TNM classification of cancer staging designated by the American Joint Committee on Cancer (AJCC)

Primary tumor (T stage)			
Tis:	Carcinoma in situ		
T1:	Invasion of lamina propria or submucosa		
T2:	Invasion of muscularis propria		
T3:	Invasion of serosa		
T4:	Invasion of adjacent structures		
Lymph node status (N stage)			
N0:	No local or regional lymph node involvement		
N1:	Metastases to 1–6 regional lymph nodes		
N2:	Metastases to 7–15 regional lymph nodes		
N3:	Metastases to more than 15 regional lymph nodes		
Metastatic disease (M stage)			
M0:	No distant metastases		
M1:	Distant metastases present		
Stage			
0	Tis	N0	M0
IA	T1	N0	M0
IB	T1	N1	M0
	T2	N0	M0
II	T1	N2	M0
	T2	N1	M0
	T3	N0	M0
IIIA	T2	N2	M0
	T3	N1	M0
	T4	N0	M0
IIIB	T3	N2	M0
IV	T4	N1–3	M0
	T1–3	N3	M0
	T1–4	N0–2	M1

3 cm away from the primary tumor; and N3 indicates more distant intra-abdominal lymph node involvement (duodenal, mesenteric, para-aortic, and retropancreatic) that is usually more difficult to resect surgically [22, 23, 24].

The International Union Against Cancer (UICC) has developed a new staging system for N stage (Figure 7.5) which relies on the number of positive lymph nodes rather than their location. N0 indicates no lymph node metastases; N1 denotes

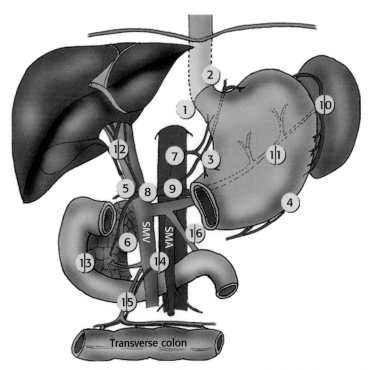

Figure 7.4. Regional lymph nodes of the stomach according to the Japanese Research Society for Gastric Cancer. 1 = right pericardium, 2 = left pericardium, 3 = lesser curvature, 4 = greater curvature, 5 = suprapyloric, 6 = infrapyloric, 7 = left gastric artery, 8 = common hepatic artery, 9 = celiac artery, 10 = splenic hilum, 11 = proximal splenic artery, 12 = hepatoduodenal ligament, 13 = retropancreatic, 14 = superior mesenteric root, 15 = middle colic vessels, 16 = para-aortic. SMA = superior mesenteric artery; SMV = superior mesenteric vein. From Lim JS, Yun MJ, Kim M-J *et al.* CT and PET in stomach cancer: preoperative staging and monitoring of response to therapy. *Radiographics* 26 (2006), 143–56. Figure 3, page 144.

metastases in 1–6 regional lymph nodes; N2 indicates metastases in 7–15 regional lymph nodes; N3 denotes metastases in greater than 15 regional lymph nodes. This new staging system correlates with clinical outcome better than the previous AJCC N criteria, with a more significant difference in survival between each N group and less deviation within the N1 and N2 groups [22, 23, 24].

The Japanese Research Society for Gastric Cancer classifies the regional lymph nodes surrounding the stomach into four compartments. These compartments determine the extent of lymph node dissection (D1–D4). Compartment I includes the perigastric lymph nodes, stations 1–6. Compartment II contains lymph nodes along the left gastric artery (station 7) and common hepatic artery (station 8), around the celiac axis (station 9), at the splenic hilum (station 10), and along the splenic

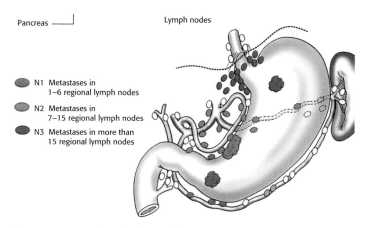

Pancreas

Lymph nodes

N1 Metastases in
1–6 regional lymph nodes

N2 Metastases in
7–15 regional lymph nodes

N3 Metastases in more than
15 regional lymph nodes

Figure 7.5. International Union Against Cancer staging system for N-stage disease relies on the number of positive nodes rather than their location. From McLean A. Gastric cancer. In Husband JE and Reznek RH eds. *Imaging in Oncology*, 2nd edn. London: Taylor and Francis, 2004; pp. 189–216, Figure 11.1, p. 192.

artery (station 11). Compartment III includes lymph nodes in the hepatoduodenal ligament (station 12), at the posterior aspect of the pancreatic head (station 13), and at the root of the mesentery (station 14). Lymph nodes along the splenic artery are considered compartment III nodes for tumors which arise in the lower third of the stomach. Compartment IV nodes include lymph nodes along the middle colic vessels (station 15) and the para-aortic lymph nodes (station 16) [22, 23, 24].

In patients undergoing a D1 lymph node dissection, the perigastric nodes attached directly to the stomach (compartment I) are removed. A D2 lymphadenectomy entails complete dissection of compartments I and II, as is the standard surgical procedure for gastric cancer in high-prevalence countries such as Japan and Korea. D3 resection involves removal of compartments I–III. D4 lymphadenectomy removes all four compartments. According to the new AJCC classification system, regional lymph nodes of stations 12–16 are classified as distant metastases (M1). Accordingly, detailed anatomic nodal descriptions based on lymph node location remain an important component of preoperative nodal staging [30, 31].

Adequate surgical resection (R0) is the only potentially curative therapy for eligible patients with gastric cancer. In the West, gastric cancer is often diagnosed at an advanced stage of disease that is not eligible for surgery. Fewer than 50% of patients undergo R0 resection.

New concepts of multimodality treatment strategies for locally advanced gastric carcinoma have been investigated. Several Phase II and III clinical trials for neoadjuvant chemotherapy in gastric carcinoma have shown its feasibility and safety. Its purpose is to eliminate or delay systemic metastasis and reduce micrometastatic spread of disease. Another benefit is potential reduction of tumor volume in initially unresectable advanced tumor stages (down-staging), therefore increasing resectability rates. An adequate treatment strategy, especially regarding the concept of neoadjuvant chemotherapy, requires precise clinical staging to predict relevant prognostic factors and identify resectable tumor stages [30, 31].

Patterns of tumor spread

Gastric cancer spreads beyond the confines of the stomach via a variety of routes: direct extension, intraperitoneal seeding, lymphangitic invasion, and hematogenous metastases. Knowledge of the usual pathways of dissemination is helpful in predicting the location of and detecting the presence of metastases on cross-sectional imaging studies.

Direct invasion
The mesenteric reflections and ligaments provide an important natural pathway for direct extension of gastric cancer into the liver, colon, pancreas and spleen.

Lesser omentum
The superior aspect of the lesser omentum is composed of the gastrohepatic ligament and inferiorly it consists of the hepatoduodenal ligament. The gastrohepatic ligament extends between the lesser curvature of the stomach and the liver, attached in its upper portion deep within the ligamentum venosum and more inferiorly within the porta hepatis. The subperitoneal areolar tissue of the gastrohepatic ligament continues into the liver as Glisson's capsule. The vascular landmarks of the gastrohepatic ligament are the left gastric artery and vein and the right gastric artery and vein that form an anastomotic arcade along the lesser curvature of the stomach. It also contains the left gastric lymph node chain. It forms the barrier between the left peritoneal space and the lesser sac. The free edge of the gastrohepatic ligament, which extends from the flexure between the first and second portions of the duodenum to the porta hepatis, envelops the hepatic artery, portal vein, bile duct, and lymph nodes of the porta hepatis. The lesser omentum is a frequent site of tumor invasion from gastric (Figures 7.6 and 7.7) and esophageal cancers as well as those arising from the gastroesophageal junction [30, 31, 32, 33, 34, 35].

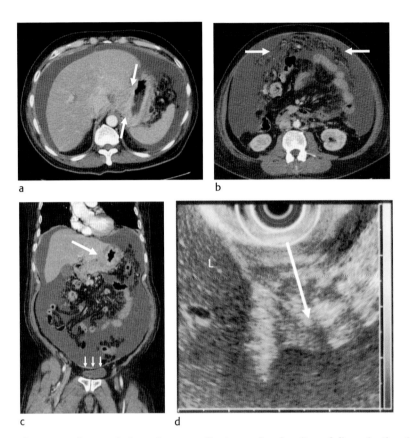

Figure 7.6a–d. Spread of gastric cancer: direct spread and peritoneal dissemination. (a) Axial CT image shows a tumor of the proximal stomach extending into the gastrohepatic ligament (arrows). (b) Scan obtained more inferiorly reveals tumor implants in the greater omentum (arrows). Note the large amount of ascites in both images. (c) Coronal multiplanar reformatted (MPR) image shows tumor in the gastrohepatic ligament (large arrow) and peritoneal implants in the pelvis (small arrows). (d) Endoscopic ultrasound (EUS) image showing invasion of perigastric fat (arrow). L = liver.

Gastrocolic ligament

The gastrocolic ligament extends inferiorly from the greater curvature of the stomach to suspend the transverse colon. It extends anteriorly and inferiorly as an apron to become the greater omentum, which covers the colon and small bowel in the peritoneal cavity. On the left, the gastrocolic ligament is contiguous with the gastrosplenic ligament and on the right it is fused with the transverse mesocolon. It is inserted and attached to the retroperitoneum behind the pylorus and anterior to the head of the pancreas. The vascular landmarks of the gastrocolic ligament are the left and right gastroepiploic vessels that course along the greater curvature of the stomach [30, 31, 32, 33, 34, 35].

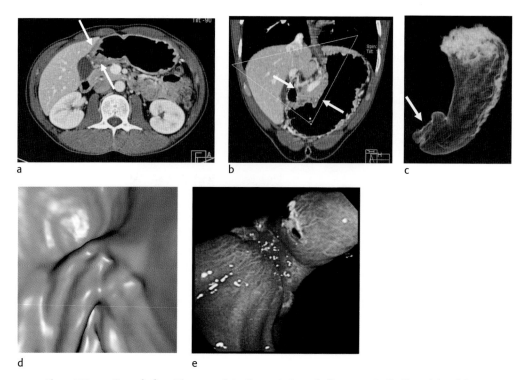

a   b   c

d   e

Figure 7.7a–e. Spread of gastric cancer into the gastrohepatic ligament: CT findings. (a) Axial CT scan shows mural thickening of the gastric antrum (arrows) with loss of mural stratification. (b) Coronal MPR image demonstrates tumor growing into the gastrohepatic ligament (arrows). (c) Shaded surface display image depicts distortion of the gastric contour (arrow). Virtual gastroscopy (VG) image (d) and endoscopic views (e) show an elevated lesion along the lesser curvature of the antrum.

Gastric lesions that extend down the subperitoneal space of the gastrocolic ligament (Figure 7.8) typically involve the superior haustral row of the transverse colon, which becomes fixed and straightened with selective loss of haustral sacculations [30, 31, 32, 33, 34, 35].

Gastrosplenic ligament

The gastrosplenic ligament connects the posterolateral wall of the fundus and greater curvature of the stomach to the splenic hilum. It forms the lateral boundary of the lesser sac. The vascular landmarks of the gastrosplenic ligament include the short gastric artery and vein at the fundus and the segments of the left gastroepiploic artery and vein branching from the splenic artery and vein at the hilum of the spleen along the body of the stomach. Cancers of the greater curvature of the

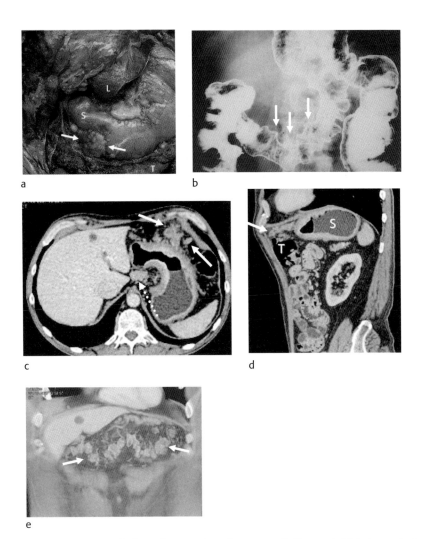

Figure 7.8a–e. Spread of gastric cancer into the gastrocolic ligament. (a) Autopsy photograph shows tumor (arrows) extending from the gastric antrum (S) into the transverse colon (T) via the gastrocolic ligament. L = liver. (b) Double contrast barium enema shows invasion along the superior aspect of the transverse colon (arrows). In a different patient axial (c), sagittal MPR (d), coronal MPR (e) images show tumor invading the gastrocolic ligament (solid arrows) and gastrohepatic ligament (discontinuous arrows in c).

gastric body and fundus typically recruit this pathway (Figure 7.9). The subperitoneal space of this ligament is also continuous with the splenorenal ligament, which allows spread of disease between the stomach, spleen, and tail of the pancreas [30, 31, 32, 33, 34, 35].

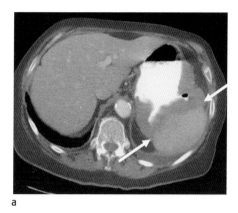
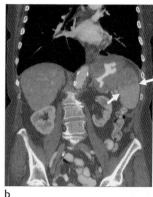

a   b

Figure 7.9a,b. Spread of gastric cancer into the splenic hilum via the subperitoneal space of the gastrosplenic ligament. Axial CT scan (a) and coronal MPR image (b) demonstrate gastric cancer invading the gastrosplenic ligament and splenic hilum (arrows).

Lymphatic invasion

Gastric cancer commonly invades adjacent lymphatics, and identification of specific nodal groups is an important part of the staging process (Figures 7.10 and 7.11). These metastases generally follow lymphatic pathways in the adjacent peritoneal ligaments, subperitoneal spaces, mesenteries, and omenta. The pathways of lymphatic drainage accompany the blood vessels supplying or draining the stomach. Lymphatic tumor emboli however are not always arrested in the nearest draining lymph node. Lymphatic obstruction of a more remote node may occur because of cellular impaction. This can cause retrograde tumor spread to an adjacent segment of gut or a more distant portion of the alimentary tract [30, 31, 32, 33, 34, 35].

Hematogenous metastases

Gastric cancers shed as many as 4 million cells per gram of tumor tissue into the bloodstream every day [36]. The vast majority are rapidly cleared from the circulation. Despite this metastatic inefficiency, the liver and gut are common sites of hematogenous metastases (Figure 7.12). The portal vein is the major conduit of tumor cells to the liver, which is particularly vulnerable to the deposition of metastases due to its architecture. Metastases extravasate through the fenestrations in the sinusoids and receive a rich mixture of arterial and portal venous blood. In this favorable milieu, it is not surprising that hepatic metastases may grow four to six times faster than metastases at other sites. Less common sites of hematogenous metastases include the lungs, adrenal glands, and skeleton [37].

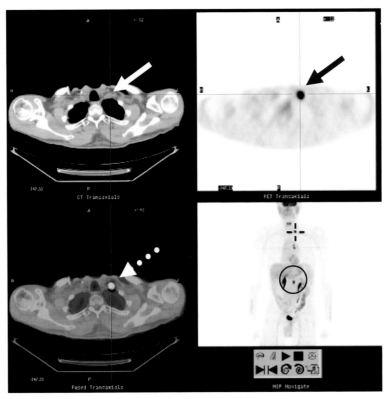

Figure 7.10. Lymphatic spread of gastric cancer: Virchow's node. PET-CT scan shows increased metabolic activity in a left supraclavicular lymph node on the CT image (solid white arrow), the FDG-PET (solid black arrow) image, and the axial fused image (discontinuous white arrow). The gastric primary neoplasm (circle) is visualized on the coronal FDG-PET image.

Peritoneal seeding

The spread of malignant gastric tumor cells in the peritoneal cavity is determined by a number of factors: the presence of ligaments, mesenteries, and omenta; intraperitoneal fluid pressure gradients; cell type and mitotic rate; and the presence of adhesions and previous surgery. Malignant gastric cells grow where natural flow allows the affected ascites to pool (Figure 7.13). Malignant cells and fluid in the inframesocolic space seek the pelvis but may first deposit on the superior aspect of the sigmoid colon on the left and the medial aspect of the cecum on the right. In the pelvis, these malignant cells fill the pouch of Douglas and then the paravesical recesses. Malignant pelvic fluid then ascends both paracolic gutters, driven by negative intra-abdominal pressure associated with breathing and the topography of peritoneal recesses. Flow of malignant fluid in the left paracolic gutter is modest and limited by the phrenicocolic

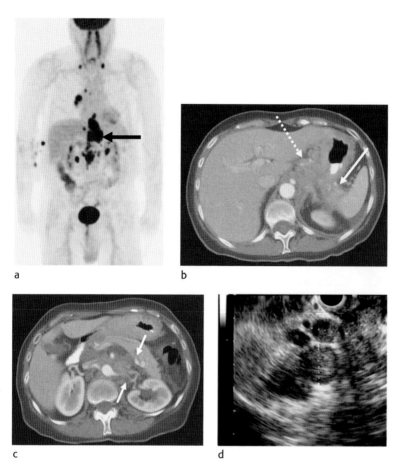

a   b

c   d

Figure 7.11a–d. Lymphatic tumor spread on PET, MDCT, and EUS. (a) Multiple mediastinal, supraclavicular, and retroperitoneal lymph nodes show increased metabolic activity on PET scan due to metastatic involvement by the patient's primary neoplasm (arrow). (b) CT scan shows tumor invasion of the gastrohepatic ligament (discontinuous arrow), the gastrosplenic ligament (solid arrow), and ascites lateral to the spleen. (c) CT scan obtained caudal to (b) shows retroperitoneal adenopathy (arrows). (d) EUS in a different patient shows enlarged celiac lymph nodes (caliper markings) due to metastatic involvement.

ligament. Most flow occurs in the right paracolic gutter, which communicates with Morison's pouch, the right subphrenic space, and potentially the lesser sac through the anterior subhepatic space and the epiploic foramen of Winslow. Seeded peritoneal metastases most commonly occur in the pouch of Douglas, the lower small bowel mesentery near the ileocecal junction, the sigmoid mesocolon, the right paracolic gutter, and the right subhepatic and right subphrenic spaces [32, 33, 38, 39].

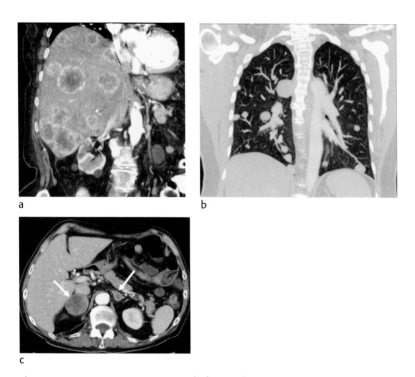

a   b

c

Figure 7.12a–c. Hematogenous spread of tumor from gastric cancer in three different patients on MDCT. (a) Coronal MPR CT image shows multiple hepatic metastases with peripheral enhancement. (b) Coronal MPR CT image demonstrates multiple pulmonary metastases. (c) Axial image shows bilateral adrenal metastases.

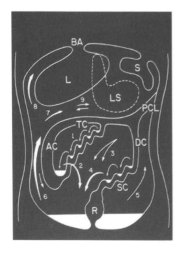

Figure 7.13. Pathways of peritoneal tumor spread. Fluid in the right inframesocolic space (1) cascades down the leaves of the small bowel mesentery, pools at the medial aspect of the cecum, and then overflows into the pelvis (2). Fluid in the left inframesocolic space (3) seeks the pelvis directly or is deposited on the superior aspect of the sigmoid mesocolon and then flows into the pelvis (4). Fluid in the pelvis may ascend the left paracolic gutter (5) but is stopped by the phrenicocolic ligament (PCL). Fluid in the right paracolic gutter (6) ascends to Morison's pouch (7) and then to the subphrenic space (8), where it is stopped at the bare area (BA) of the liver (L). There is potential communication with the lesser sac (LS) through the foramen of Winslow (9). AC = ascending colon; DC = descending colon; R = rectum; S = spleen; SC = sigmoid colon; TC = transverse colon.

The peritoneal reflections differ in the proximal and distal portions of the stomach and this has important implications for tumor dissemination. The visceral peritoneum covers the gastric surface except for a small posterior–inferior area, near the cardia, where the stomach contacts the diaphragm at the reflections of the gastrophrenic and left gastropancreatic folds. This so-called "gastric bare area" encroaches upon the posterior surface of the gastric fundus and subcardinal portion between the right and left layers of the gastrophrenic ligament, and lies between the superior and splenic recesses of the lesser sac. These portions of the stomach are actually extraperitoneal with no visceral peritoneum or serosa. Accordingly, proximal gastric cancers can invade the gastric bare area and subsequently the retroperitoneum. The partial extraperitoneal location of the proximal stomach allows lymphatic spread towards the gastric bare area, para-aortic region, left renal vein, left renal hilum, and splenic hilum [35].

Ovarian involvement (Figure 7.14), also known as Krukenberg tumors, may occur via three pathways: hematogenous spread, peritoneal dissemination, and lymphatic invasion.

Multidetector computed tomography (MDCT)

Recent improvements in MDCT technology allow thinner collimation and faster scanning. These hardware developments coupled with advances in three-dimensional imaging software and the availability of cheaper data storage capacity

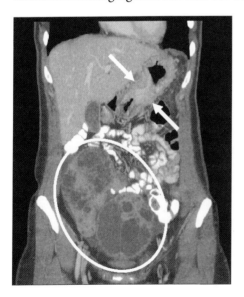

Figure 7.14. Peritoneal spread of tumor: Krukenberg tumor. Coronal reformatted CT scan shows a gastric neoplasm with mural thickening (arrows). Note the large bilateral pelvic masses (white circle) which proved to be metastases from a primary gastric adenocarcinoma to the ovaries.

have provided new opportunities for imaging the stomach and other portions of the GI tract. Isotropic imaging of the stomach is now possible providing two-dimensional multiplanar reformations (MPR), virtual gastroscopy (VG), shaded surface display images, and transparency rendering from a single data acquisition [40, 41, 42, 43, 44, 45, 46, 47, 48, 49, 50, 51, 52, 53, 54, 55, 56, 57, 58, 59, 60, 61, 62, 63, 64, 65, 66, 67, 68, 69, 70, 71, 72, 73, 74].

Dedicated gastric imaging with MDCT requires adequate gastric distention. If the entire stomach is not distended, disease may be missed and a partially collapsed stomach may mimic disease. There are two primary means of distending the stomach, with either gas or water.

Gas distension

Gastric distension can be obtained with the administration of 6 g of effervescent granules with a small amount of water after a 6-h fast. The patient is then placed in the prone position and a scout image is taken to ensure adequate gastric distention. The entire stomach is scanned without intravenous contrast material. The patient is then turned into the supine position and a second scanogram is obtained to assure gastric distention. A second dose of crystals may be given if the stomach is not optimally distended.

The stomach is scanned in the supine position with intravenous contrast material at a rate of 3 or 4 ml/s. Staging gastric cancer is better determined with intravascular contrast enhancement and the scans are performed during the portal venous phase, approximately 70 s following the injection of contrast material. If CT angiography is to be performed, images should be obtained during the early arterial phase as well.

Water distention

After a 6-h fast, the patient ingests 500 ml of water to distend the stomach and is scanned in the prone position to prevent artifacts caused by gastric air. Patients with lesions in the cardia or fundus are scanned in the supine position. For most patients, scanning in the supine position is adequate provided there is sufficient gastric distention. If the patient has a known distal gastric tumor, there is some advantage of scanning in the prone position with gas distention to minimize artifacts from air/water interfaces. With gas distention, scanning in the left posterior oblique position provides the best means of distending the distal part of the stomach and minimizing residual fluid [43].

Laparoscopic-assisted distal gastrectomy with lymph node dissection is becoming an increasingly popular method of treating EGC because it requires smaller surgical incisions, and has less intraoperative blood loss, faster recovery of normal bowel function, and shorter hospital stays than in the case of conventional open surgery. Laparoscopic gastrectomy is a technically challenging procedure because it is difficult to obtain an image of the entire view of the operative field under the laparoscope; also, the lesion, organs, and vessels cannot be directly manipulated. Since vascular preservation is necessary, a more detailed understanding of local anatomy is required during laparoscopic surgery compared with open conventional surgery. The branching patterns and morphology of the blood vessels are more complex in the stomach than in the colon and it is useful to preoperatively identify the right gastric artery, the left gastric artery, and left gastric vein for laparoscopically assisted gastrectomy [43]. Several studies have proven the utility of MDCT angiography and venography in these patients [44, 45].

T staging

The normal stomach distended with gas or water typically measures less than 6 mm in thickness. The gastric antrum is usually thicker than the gastric body or fundus. Pickhardt and Asher found that the distal antrum has a mean thickness of 5.1 ± 1.6 mm and mural stratification, with a lower density submucosa in 24% of patients. In the same study, the mean anterior gastric body wall thickness was 2.0 ± 0.4 mm [51].

When scanned in the axial plane, the gastroesophageal junction may also appear slightly thicker as well. Following the intravenous administration of contrast material, the gastric wall, particularly in the region of the gastric antrum, may be seen as a three-layered structure, with maximal enhancement of the inner mucosal layer. Fat deposition may be seen in the submucosa and the outer soft tissue layer representing the muscularis propria and serosal layer. The serosal margin of the stomach is usually well defined, highlighted against the low-density perigastric fat.

On MDCT, AGCs manifest with mural thickening and abnormal mucosal enhancement. EGC can be less reliably visualized but detection is improved with VG and MPR techniques. The imaging features depend on the histologic type of tumor and the size and depth of invasion [52].

A high degree of contrast enhancement is significantly more common in signet ring cancer (SRC) than non-SRC. This pattern is secondary to the well-known differences in contrast enhancement between mature and immature fibrotic tissue. Groups of signet ring cells intermingled with immature and loose fibrotic tissue induce a high degree of enhancement. Mature scar (fibrotic tissue) is composed mainly of dense collagen fibers but few cells and vessels, whereas early or immature fibrotic tissue contains abundant fibroblasts and neovascularity. As a consequence, mature fibrotic tissue shows poor contrast enhancement whereas early or immature fibrotic tissue shows good contrast enhancement during portal venous phase imaging [52].

Rossi and coworkers [53] found differences in the enhancement patterns between the two major types of gastric cancer. In diffuse gastric cancer, clusters of tumor cells infiltrate the gastric layers so that desmoplastic reaction and inflammatory peritumoral reaction are limited to the gastric wall. In these patients, mural stratification may be maintained with a hyperdense inner wall and hypodense outer wall. A smooth and regular appearance of the outer wall is typical of T1 and T2 lesions. In intestinal gastric cancer, cells are more closely linked and organized in solid and glandular structures that replace the gastric layers completely. In these cases, mural stratification is lost as desmoplasia and necrosis distort the outer gastric wall.

Initial reports found close agreement between T staging as determined by CT and pathologic staging. Subsequent reports have been less sanguine so that EUS is currently the most reliable method for preoperative determination of earlier T stage disease [2].

On CT, in the presence of T1 and T2 lesions (Figures 7.15, 7.16 and 7.17) in which invasion is limited to the gastric wall, the outer border of the stomach is typically smooth. With T3 lesions (Figure 7.18), the serosal contours become blurred and strand-like areas of increased density are often seen extending into the perigastric fat. In T4 lesions (Figures 7.19 and 7.20), there is frank tumor extension into the subperitoneal spaces of the various ligaments and omenta and subsequently adjacent organs

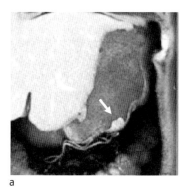 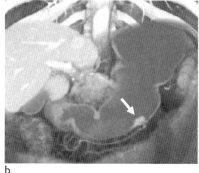

a   b

Figure 7.15a,b. Type I early gastric cancer on MDCT. Coronal MPR images (a, b) obtained with a fluid-distended stomach show a mass along the greater curvature of the stomach (arrows).

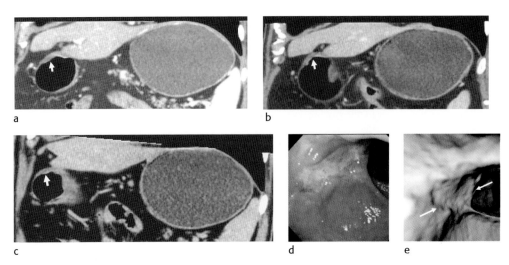

Figure 7.16a–e. T1, N0 carcinoma of the gastric antrum (arrows). Coronal MPR images obtained 40 s (a), 70 s (b), and 150 s (c) following the intravenous administration of contrast material show focal mural thickening along the lesser curvature aspect of the stomach. Upper GI endoscopy (d) and VG (e) views of this antral neoplasm (arrows).

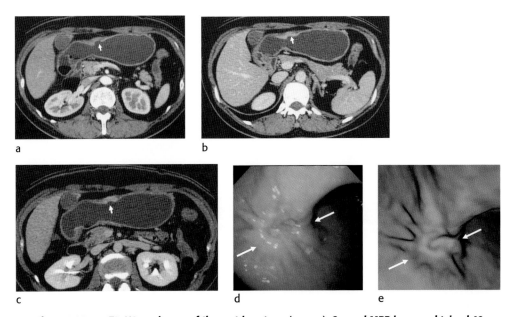

Figure 7.17a–e. T2, N0 carcinoma of the gastric antrum (arrows). Coronal MPR images obtained 40 s (a), 70 s (b), and 150 s (c) following the intravenous administration of contrast material show a type III ulcerating mass along the lesser curvature aspect of the gastric angulus. Upper GI endoscopy (d) and VG (e) images of this early gastric cancer (arrows).

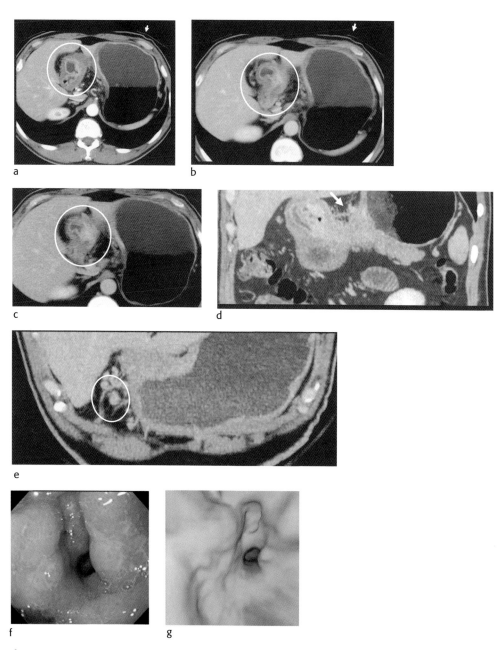

Figure 7.18a–g. T3, N1 carcinoma of the gastric antrum. Axial images obtained 40 s (a), 70 s (b), and 150 s (c) following the intravenous administration of contrast material depict this circumferential antral neoplasm (circles). (d) Coronal MPR image shows prominent perigastric fat infiltration (arrow) on this scan obtained at 70 s. (e) Coronal MPR image demonstrates perigastric metastatic lymphadenopathy (circle). Upper GI endoscopy (f) and VG (g) views of this advanced gastric cancer.

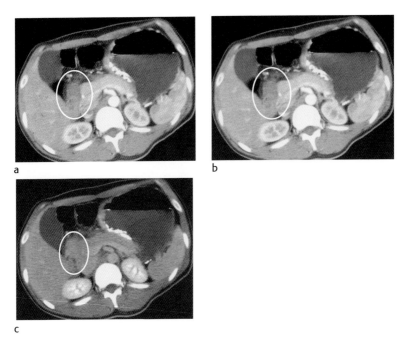

Figure 7.19a–c. T4 carcinoma of the gastric antrum (circles) invading the pancreas. Axial CT images obtained 40 s (a), 70 s (b), and 150 s (c) following the intravenous administration of contrast material show a poorly marginated antral mass that invades the pancreatic head.

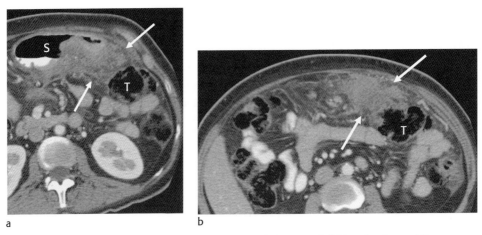

Figure 7.20a,b. T4 carcinoma of the greater curvature of the stomach (S) invades (arrows) the transverse colon (T) on these axial MDCT images.

and/or into the peritoneal cavity. The spleen may be invaded via the gastrosplenic ligament, the liver via the lesser omentum, the pancreas via the lesser sac.

It is very important to differentiate between T3 and T4 lesions because invasion of adjacent structures makes surgery very difficult. If a gastric mass abuts an adjacent organ on CT and there is absence of a fat plane between the mass and the organ, tumor invasion should be suspected, but this finding is not diagnostic for invasion.

In one study [54], the accuracy of 64-channel MDCT for the detection of gastric cancer was 90% for EGC and 100% for AGC, with an overall detection rate of 95%. Accuracy for detection of T stage was 89% for EGC and 88% for AGC, with an overall accuracy of 88%. Its accuracy for determining lymph node metastases was 90% for EGC and 71% for AGC, with an overall accuracy of 80%.

A number of studies employing MPR images have shown improved accuracy when compared to axial images alone [50]. Using the water-filling method, Shimizu *et al.* [55] found that MPR added value in the staging of gastric cancer. The detection rate of all gastric cancers was 65%, with a detection rate of 96.2% for AGC and 41.2% for EGC. Kim *et al.* [56] found isotropic MDCT with MPR images including coronal and sagittal reconstructions improved the accuracy of preoperative T and N staging for AGC with little impact on the accuracy of staging EGC. In another study, Hur and coworkers [57] demonstrated that MPR images enabled more accurate preoperative T staging of gastric cancer but there was no improvement in N staging. T stage accuracy of axial and combined axial and MPR images was 67% versus 77%. In one study, Kim and others [56] found that the overall N staging accuracy was 54% versus 59% for T staging, which was not significantly different. Gastric cancer was detected in 87% of patients with axial CT images and in 98% using volumetric CT imaging. The overall accuracy of tumor staging was 77% with transverse CT imaging and 84% with volumetric CT imaging. The overall accuracy for lymph node staging was 62% with transverse CT imaging and 64% with volumetric CT imaging. For staging metastases, there was no difference in accuracy between transverse and volumetric CT imaging.

In a study comparing 3D MDCT and upper GI series, Chen and coworkers [59] reported that both techniques had 100% accuracy in detecting the lesion. The diagnostic accuracies of MDCT and upper GI series were similar for differentiating between mucosal and submucosal lesions (94% vs 96%) as well as for classification of the Bormann type of AGC (70% vs 63%). MDCT had an accuracy of 73% in T staging and 69% in N staging.

In assessing serosal invasion by gastric cancer, Kumano *et al.* [60] found that MDCT had 93% accuracy, with scirrhous subtypes of carcinomas more frequently understaged.

N staging

On MDCT, as in MRI, the diagnosis of adenopathy depends upon size criteria based on short-axis diameter. Lymph nodes in the upper abdomen vary between 6 and 11 mm depending on their location. Lymph nodes in the gastrohepatic ligament are considered abnormal if they exceed 8 mm in diameter [61]. Lymph node size is not a reliable indicator of lymph node metastases in patients with gastric cancer. In a study of 1253 lymph nodes in 31 surgical specimens, 74% were tumor free and 26% contained metastases. The mean diameter of tumor-free nodes was 4.1 mm, whereas tumor-containing nodes had a mean diameter of 6.0 mm. Of tumor-free lymph nodes, 80% were smaller than 5 mm, whereas 55% of nodes containing metastases were less than 5 mm in size. Seven of ten patients without lymph node metastases had at least one node larger than 10 mm and 15 of 21 patients with lymph node metastases had a least one node that was 10 mm or greater in diameter [61].

M staging

Liver metastases are present in up to 25% of patients with AGC at the time of presentation although liver metastases are unusual in patients with EGC. The presence of ascites usually indicates peritoneal seeding although depiction of an individual, small peritoneal deposit may be beneath the spatial resolution of CT. Laparoscopy is more sensitive than CT in the detection of small peritoneal deposits.

Gastric cancer is one of the most common malignancies to metastasize to the ovaries. Approximately 5%–20% of ovarian cancers are metastatic lesions. Ovarian metastases precede the detection of the primary site in 38% of cases. Most Krukenberg tumors are solid tumors that contain well demarcated intramural cysts that demonstrate robust contrast enhancement. In comparison with ovarian metastases from colon cancer, gastric metastases tend to be smaller, appear more solid, and more frequently have dense enhancement of the solid component [62].

Endoscopic ultrasound

Since the late 1990s EUS has been used as a standard to preoperatively stage patients at high risk of recurrence for enrollment in neoadjuvant protocols. Patients with locoregionally advanced disease are at significant risk for recurrence and death after complete resection. Although postoperative adjuvant chemoradiation can reduce this risk, it does not eliminate it. Furthermore, postoperative adjuvant chemoradiation therapy is quite difficult to tolerate. Combined assessment of serosal invasion and nodal positivity on EUS identifies 77% of those at risk for death from gastric cancer after curative resection [75]. Combined assessment of depth of tumor penetration and nodal positivity on EUS not only has the highest concordance with pathology but also identifies patients at the highest risk for death from gastric cancer [76].

Endoscopic US has become a primary means of locoregional staging of gastric carcinoma. By virtue of its ability to depict five major layers in the gastric wall, which correspond to histologic layers, EUS can determine the depth of tumor invasion and the involvement of regional lymph nodes. EUS has added greatly to the staging of gastric cancers but there are some limitations not found with esophageal cancer. Problems may arise in distinguishing the muscularis propria from the serosa when trying to define a gastric lesion as T2 or T3. For cancers limited to the mucosa, EUS confers significant advantages over CT and with the advent of EMR (endoscopic mucosal resection) for EGC, appropriate staging of gastric cancer limited to the mucosa or invading the muscularis mucosa is very important. Combination of EUS and EMR for EGC appears very promising. For infiltrating gastric malignancies, EUS is also helpful in assessing the extent of disease [77, 78, 79, 80, 81, 82, 83, 84].

Instrumentation and techniques

Endoscopic US (Figure 7.21) combines features of endoscopy and ultrasound in two major types of echoendoscope. A standard endoscopic exam is performed before the EUS to localize the gastric lesion. The echoendoscope is passed into the

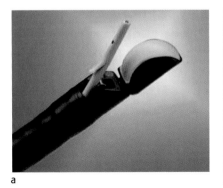

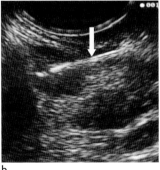

a   b

Figure 7.21a,b. Sonoendoscope. (a) Linear echoendoscopes use an electronic curved-array transducer mounted in front of the optical lens of an oblique viewing endoscope. (b) These sonoendoscopes have the ability to biopsy masses and suspicious lymph nodes. A biopsy needle (arrow) is visualized on this endosonogram.

stomach and the transducer is placed perpendicular to the gastric wall. The balloon is inflated, gastric air is removed, and the stomach is then filled with deaerated water. The scope is moved back and forth to evaluate the extent of the tumor, the layer of origin, and lymph node involvement. Two major types of endoscope are employed: radial endoscopes and linear endoscopes. Both probes achieve acoustic coupling with the stomach by filling a latex balloon covering the transducer with deaerated water or by placing 300–500 ml of water into the intestinal lumen. With the incorporation of color flow and Doppler data, the utility of this technique has expanded [83].

A number of frequencies can be used while performing EUS. A lower-frequency transducer (7.5 MHz) provides visualization of organs and lesions extrinsic to the gastric wall. While a 12-MHz transducer nicely depicts the gastric wall, a 20-MHz transducer provides the highest mural resolution but has a depth of penetration limited to 15 mm [83].

Radial echoendoscopes

These instruments use a built-in mechanical or electronic rotating transducer that is rotated in a 360-degree arc by a motor mounted in the proximal portion of the endoscope. This produces a radial sonographic image that is perpendicular to the long axis of the endoscope. Endoscopic images can be obtained simultaneously, but the angle of view is 80° oblique to the image obtained with the standard viewing endoscope. Current radial endoscopes have the capability to switch from frequencies of 5 to 20 MHz to optimize depth of penetration and image resolution. The higher frequencies provide superb mural imaging but only provide 2 cm of tissue penetration. The lower frequencies have a depth of penetration of 8 cm and are useful for detecting extramural pathology. The radial echoendoscope is limited because it cannot follow the needle path during fine-needle aspiration [83].

Linear echoendoscopes

This instrument uses an electronic curved-array transducer mounted in front of the optical lens of an oblique viewing endoscope. It generates a 100- to 180-degree linear sector scan that is parallel to the long axis of the scope and is oriented at an angle of 90° to the radial anatomy. Linear probes can generate color flow and Doppler images and have a frequency range of 5 to 10 MHz. This probe is used when performing fine-needle aspiration because the needle can be tracked over its entire course from exiting the probe channel and entering and aspirating the target lesion [83].

Fine-needle aspiration

Fine-needle aspiration guided by EUS has become an important tool in the diagnosis of deep mural gastric malignancies and for providing cytologic material when assessing a lymph node. The needle course and biopsy technique depend on three factors: the size and consistency of the target lesion; the proximity of surrounding blood vessels; and the consistency of the gastric wall. The needle is advanced through the biopsy channel and is monitored with real-time sonography as it advances into the lesion [83].

Normal EUS appearance of the stomach

The normal gastric wall has five layers (Figure 7.22). The first, inner layer is hyperechoic and represents the acoustic interface between the lumen and the gastric epithelium. The second layer is hypoechoic and is composed of the deep mucosa, lamina propria, and muscularis mucosa. The next layer is hyperechoic and corresponds to the submucosa. The fourth layer is hypoechoic and is composed of the muscularis propria. The fifth, or outermost, layer corresponds to the serosa, or interface between the stomach wall and the surrounding tissue [83].

High-frequency ultrasound can often delineate the gastric wall as a seven- to nine-layered structure. In up to 70% of patients, the muscularis mucosa is visualized in two layers and the muscularis propria appears as a three-layered structure, with a circular layer, interface, and longitudinal layer [84].

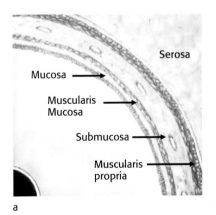
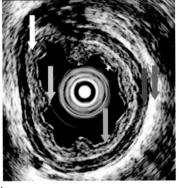

a   b

Figure 7.22a,b. Endoscopic ultrasound appearance of the normal stomach. (a) (Diagram) and (b) (EUS image) depict normal mural stratification with an echogenic inner ring (mucosa – yellow arrow), surrounded by a hypoechoic ring (muscularis mucosa – green arrow), which is surrounded by another echogenic ring (submucosa – white arrow), which is surrounded by a hypoechoic ring (muscularis propria – red arrow), which is surrounded by echogenic fat in the serosa (purple arrow).

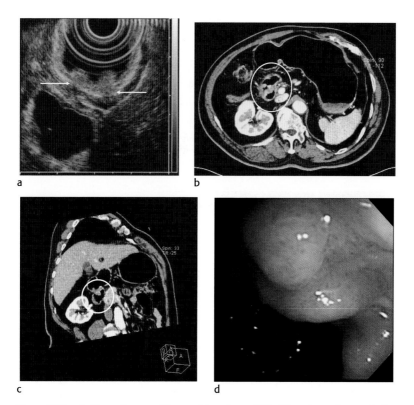

Figure 7.23a–d. T1 carcinoma of the gastric antrum: EUS, CT, endoscopic correlation.
(a) Endoscopic ultrasound shows invasion of the submucosa (arrows), however the muscularis propria is intact. Axial (b) and coronal MPR (c) CT images show the mass in the gastric antrum (circles). (d) Endoscopic view of this neoplasm.

T staging

The depth of tumor invasion is assessed by determining the disruption of the mural stratification of the stomach. EGCs are by definition limited to the mucosa and submucosa without regard to lymph node status (Figures 7.23 and 7.24). Types IIa, IIb, and IIc lesions can be identified as irregularities in the mucosal layer without involvement of the submucosa. Type III EGC shows involvement of the submucosa. On EUS, it is usually difficult to distinguish between T2 and T3 (Figures 7.25 and 7.26) lesions because the serosa may be a very thin layer or absent in some individuals. In these cases reliable determination of whether the tumor lies in the subserosa or actually penetrates the serosa may be difficult (Figure 7.27). As with CT and MRI, it is difficult for EUS to differentiate between inflammatory change and tumor. This can lead to overstaging of Stage I and Stage II tumors [75, 76, 77, 78, 79, 80, 81, 82, 83, 84].

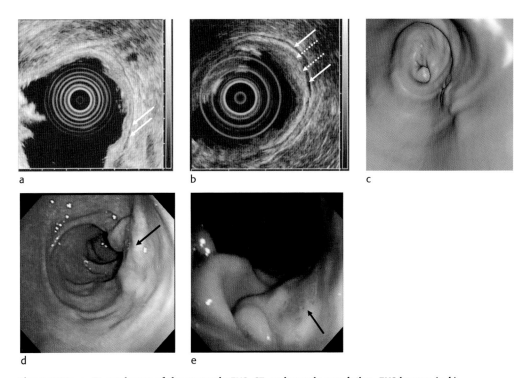

a   b   c

d   e

Figure 7.24a–e. T1 carcinoma of the stomach: EUS, CT, endoscopic correlation. EUS images (a, b) show preservation of the hypoechoic muscularis propria (solid arrows) but invasion of the submucosa (discontinuous arrows). VG (c) and upper GI endoscopy (d, e) images of this neoplasm (black arrows).

In patients with AGC, the tumor appears as an inhomogeneous, hypoechoic mass that arises from the mucosa and extends through all the layers of the gastric wall associated with loss of mural stratification. Scirrhous carcinomas may manifest as diffuse thickening of the third and fourth layers of the gastric wall with destruction of the submucosa and muscularis propria.

In a report by Yoshida and co-workers [78] the depth of EGC invasion was accurately determined in 90% of cases. The muscularis mucosa was visualized in 63% of cases. Habermann *et al.* [77], in a study comparing EUS, MDCT, and histology, found that CT achieved correct T staging in 76% and correct N staging in 70%. EUS achieved correct T staging in 86% and N staging in 90% of patients.

N staging

Endoscopic US is the most accurate means for depicting perigastric adenopathy. Nodal involvement is determined not only by size (which CT and MRI can assess) but also by morphologic characteristics of the nodes. Lymph nodes that

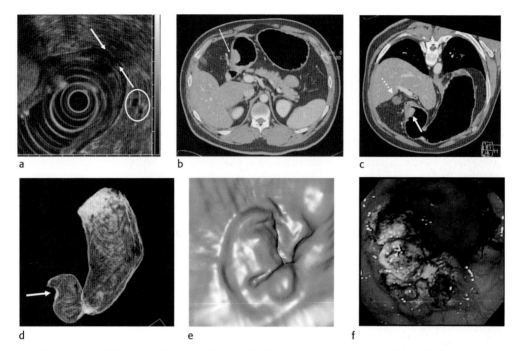

a   b   c

d   e   f

Figure 7.25a–f. T2, N1 carcinoma of the gastric antrum: EUS, CT, endoscopic correlation. (a) EUS shows tumor invading the hypoechoic muscularis propria layer (arrows). Note the spherical, small hypoechoic lymph nodes in the adjacent fat (circle). (b) Axial CT scan shows mural thickening of the lesser curvature of the antrum. Note the preserved serosal fat adjacent to the tumor (arrow). (c) MPR CT image shows the antral mass (solid arrow) and enlarged lymph node (discontinuous arrow) in the lesser omentum. (d) Shaded surface display image shows the antral mass deforming the lesser curvature (arrow). VG (e) and upper GI endoscopy (f) views of this mass.

are spherical, sharply demarcated, homogeneous, and hypoechoic indicate malignancy. Inflammatory nodes typically have poorly defined margins, are inhomogeneous and hyperechoic, and have a triangular or ellipsoid shape. Lymph nodes with micrometastases or those that measure 5 mm or less in size may be difficult to detect. With the curvilinear ultrasound probe, suspicious nodes can be biopsied, which increases the staging accuracy of this technique.

Because of the short range of ultrasound (5–7 cm), lymph nodes beyond that depth and the right lobe of the liver cannot be diagnostically visualized [75, 76, 77, 78, 79, 80, 81, 82, 83, 84].

M staging

Endoscopic US has a limited field of view and is not used for M staging. For this CT, MR, and positron emission tomography-CT (PET-CT) have a major role.

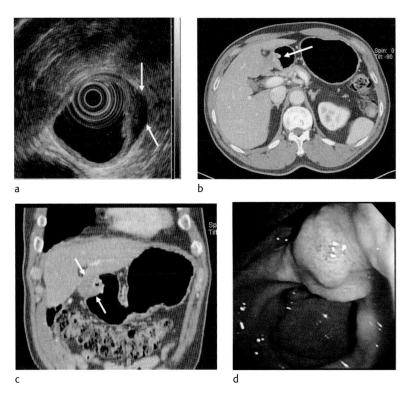

Figure 7.26a–d. **T3 carcinoma of the stomach: EUS, CT, endoscopic correlation. (a) EUS shows tumor invasion of the serosal fat (arrows). (b) Axial CT shows mural thickening of the antrum (arrow). (c) Coronal MPR image shows the mass invading the adjacent fat (arrows). (d) Upper GI endoscopic view of this tumor.**

Positron emission tomography-computed tomography (PET-CT)

Positron emission tomography became a clinical force in the mid-to-late 1990s when the US Health Care Administration approved whole-body PET imaging for several oncologic indications. The most frequently used tracer in oncology patients is the glucose analog [^{18}F]2-fluoro-2-deoxyglucose (FDG). Cellular FDG uptake is predominantly related to expression of the protein glucose transporter 1 [85, 86]. This protein is ubiquitously expressed in almost all cell types, but its overexpression in malignant tissue is quite frequent and leads to intracellular accumulation of FDG, which is visualized on PET. The high lesion-to-background contrast and whole-body data acquisition on FDG-PET represent critical advantages over CT and MRI, where contrast between pathologic and normal structures may be limited. FDG-PET has been developed to quantitatively assess local glucose metabolism. PET can

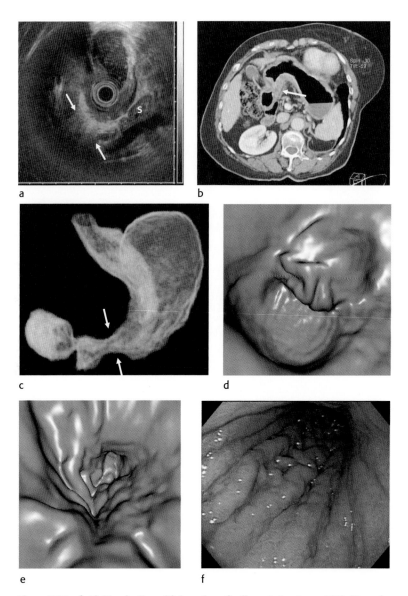

Figure 7.27a–f. Linitis plastica with invasion of adjacent structures: EUS, CT, endoscopic correlation.
(a) EUS shows diffuse mural thickening of the gastric antrum (S) with tumor invasion (arrows) of
adjacent fat. (b) MPR CT image also shows mural thickening (arrow) of the antrum. (c) Shaded surface
display image shows narrowing of the gastric antrum (arrows). VG (d, e) and upper GI endoscopy (f)
show thickening of the rugal folds.

help differentiate between benign and malignant tumors, determine the degree of malignancy, evaluate the effectiveness of chemotherapy (Figure 7.28) and/or radiotherapy, and help predict prognosis. Indeed FDG-PET has been used to screen for malignancies [85, 86].

PET-CT is a fixed combination of PET and CT scanners in a combined imaging system. The nearly simultaneous data acquisitions lead to minimization of spatial and temporal mismatches between modalities by eliminating the need to move the patient during the exam. The result is a fused image that provides biologic and anatomic information. Imaging metabolic information about tumor tissue provides often more sensitive and specific information concerning the extent of malignancy than anatomic information alone [87, 88, 89, 90].

FDG-PET is a well-accepted method for the detection and staging of a number of malignancies including lung, breast, colorectal, and esophageal cancer. FDG-PET has only assumed a secondary role in the evaluation of gastric cancer because the sensitivity of this exam for the diagnosis of primary gastric lesions, metastatic adenopathy, and peritoneal dissemination has not been stellar [91, 92, 93, 94, 95, 96, 97, 98, 99, 100, 101].

In one study [93], FDG-PET revealed increased uptake in 94% of gastric adenocarcinomas. In this series, the mean standard uptake value (SUV) was higher in AGC (7.5) than in EGC (2.1) and the sensitivity for detecting the primary tumor was 98% for AGC and 63% for EGC. The mean SUV is higher in Stages III and IV than in Stages I and II (5.4 vs 3.7) cancers. The SUV was higher in patients with tubular adenocarcinoma than in those with mucinous adenocarcinoma and SRC (7.7 vs 4.2). It is postulated that the lower uptake of these tumor types is due to the high content of metabolically inert mucus leading to a reduced FDG concentration. Another reason could be the lack of expression of the glucose transporter Glut-1 on the cell membrane of most SRCs. FDG uptake was also higher for larger tumors [91, 92, 93, 94, 95, 96, 97, 98, 99, 100, 101, 102, 103, 104, 105, 106, 107, 108, 109, 110].

To remedy the lower sensitivity of FDG uptake in certain types of gastric cancers, Herrmann *et al.* [91] reported that the pyrimidine analog 3-deoxy-3-[^{18}F]-fluorothymidine (FLT) accumulated in all local AGC irrespective of the histologic subtype. This substance has the potential to improve early evaluation of the response to neoadjuvant treatment in tumors with low FDG uptake.

T staging

PET-CT does not have a role in assessing the depth of penetration of gastric malignancies. Accurate T staging requires a high-resolution imaging modality because

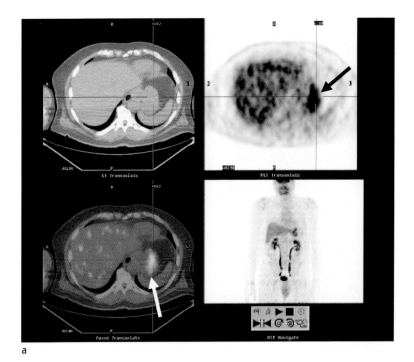

a

Figure 7.28a,b. Utility of PET-CT in evaluating therapeutic response in patients with gastric cancer. Scan obtained prior to neoadjuvant therapy (a) shows increased activity in the stomach (arrows). Following therapy (b) scans show a favorable tumor response with diminished gastric uptake of the FDG. (Cont. opposite.)

exquisite anatomic details are mandatory when deciding on the surgical resectability of primary tumors. PET-CT is better used for detecting unsuspected metastases that alter therapy [94].

The main obstacle to the routine use of FDG-PET in the management of gastric cancer is its poor sensitivity with regard to the diagnosis of the primary gastric lesion or metastatic lymph node groups [95]. The sensitivity is low because the primary gastric lesion is poorly differentiated from overlapping adjacent metastatic lymph node groups. To improve depiction of the primary tumors, Zhu et al. [89] have found that drinking 300–500 ml of milk immediately before the scan can effectively distend the stomach and increase the contrast between primary gastric tumors and the normal gastric wall. In their report, malignant lesions were observed with higher contrast and clearer outlines. The fat content in milk leads to prolonged retention of the fluid in the stomach as compared with water and provides more persistent gastric distention.

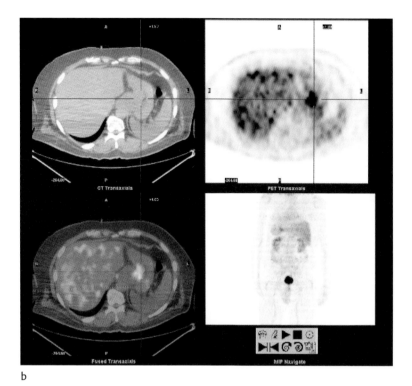

b

Figure 7.28 (Cont.)

In a study [96] of the efficacy of primary tumor assessment with PET, detection rates were significantly different in the following order: tumor size 3 cm or more (76.7%) > tumor size less than 3 cm (58.6%); AGC (82.9%) > EGC (25.9%); with nodal involvement (79.3%) > without nodal involvement (39.4%). In EGC detection of the intestinal type of cancer was 43.8% but none of the diffuse EGCs were detected. Larger or more advanced tumors with nodal involvement had a higher rate of detection by PET. In EGC only the intestinal type was detectable by PET.

N staging

The role of FDG-PET in N staging, unlike T and M staging, seems difficult to elucidate because not every lymph node can be accurately confirmed histopathologically and the evaluation of lymph nodes by individual location or number may not always be possible on FDG-PET [94]. The diagnostic performance of FDG-PET for lymph node staging is dependent on many factors including the avidity of the primary tumor for FDG, the frequency of lymph node metastases,

the size of the metastatic lymph nodes, and the prevalence of chronic inflammatory disease.

In a study [2] evaluating the utility of PET in the detection of the primary neoplasm, PET and CT showed a sensitivity of 47% for EGC and 98% for AGC. The
sensitivity of CT for N1 disease was significantly higher than that of PET. For N2
disease, PET had a sensitivity, specificity, and accuracy of 34%, 96%, and 72%
whereas the CT values were 44%, 86%, and 69%, respectively. For N3 disease, PET
and CT had a similar sensitivity, specificity, and accuracy of 50%, 99%, and 95%,
respectively. The overall sensitivity, specificity, and accuracy of PET were not significantly different than those of CT for primary tumors or for N2 and N3 metastases [2].

In another study, Chen *et al.* [93] found that FDG-PET had a significantly higher
specificity than CT (92% vs 62%) and a significantly lower sensitivity (56% vs 78%),
but similar overall accuracy (63% vs 75%) in the depiction of local lymph node
involvement. The low focal uptake of an involved lymph node may be inseparable
from that of the primary lesion, which usually has intense uptake.

Kim and coworkers [95] found that the sensitivity, specificity, positive predictive
value, and negative predictive value of FDG-PET for lymph node metastases were
40%, 95%, 91%, and 56%, respectively. SRC was associated with the lowest sensitivity (15%).

M staging

A number of studies attest to the accuracy of PET and PET-CT in the depiction of
liver metastases from a number of different primary tumors. CT however remains
the first choice for detecting peritoneal metastases (Figure 7.29) and its sensitivity is
dependent upon the size, site, and morphology of the tumor deposits, the presence
of ascites, the paucity of intra-abdominal fat, the adequacy of bowel opacification
and the concomitant use of peritoneography. CT has a higher sensitivity (76.5% vs
35.3%) and lower specificity (91.6% vs 98.9%), and an equal accuracy (89.3%) when
compared to PET imaging. CT is also superior to PET when comparing the diagnostic performance of the two modalities (91.6% vs 71.4%, respectively) [102].

There are three problems with PET that may limit sensitivity in this regard. First
is the low spatial resolution of PET, so that small seeded peritoneal nodules may
remain undetected. Secondly FDG uptake shows variable results according to cell
differentiation. Thirdly, there is marked interobserver variability for physiologic

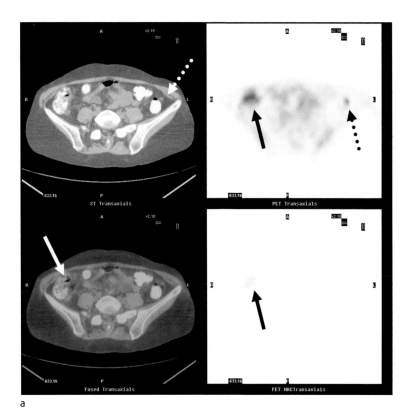

a

Figure 7.29a,b. Peritoneal recurrence of gastric cancer on PET-CT. (a) Recurrent tumor is identified along the left paracolic gutter (discontinuous arrow) and adjacent to the ascending colon (solid arrows). (b) Recurrent tumor is also visualized in the pelvis (arrows). (Cont. overleaf.)

peritoneal FDG uptake due to differences in peristalsis and involuntary muscle activity. PET-CT can minimize the limitations of both modalities.

In another study comparing PET alone with CT [93] in their ability to detect peritoneal dissemination, PET was inferior to CT. These patients tended to have small peritoneal nodules less than 5 mm in size. The pathology showed mainly extensive fibrosis with a small number of malignant cells in the disseminated lesion. The actual tumor cells were too sparse and spread out to be detectable by the PET scanner. CT had a high sensitivity in detecting peritoneal dissemination but low specificity due to high false-positive findings. When detecting peritoneal carcinomatosis, CT can readily detect peritoneal and omental caking, nodularity, beaded thickening, and malignant ascites [93].

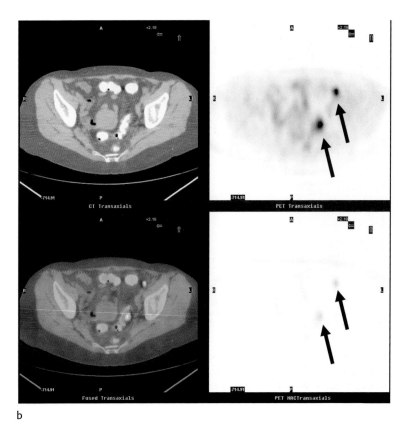

b

Figure 7.29 (Cont.)

Magnetic resonance imaging

To date, MRI (Figures 7.30 and 7.31) has not achieved a primary imaging role in the management of patients with gastric cancer. This is because of a number of limitations including motion artifacts, high costs, and the limited degree of spatial resolution afforded by standard body coils. In-vitro studies have shown that MRI allows the depiction of the gastric wall layers and technically permits the evaluation of the local tumor stage of gastric carcinomas. The results achieved by experimental MRI systems are not yet available in clinical practice [103, 104, 105, 106, 107, 108, 109, 110, 111].

As with MDCT, MRI evaluation of the stomach is best achieved with distention and hypotonia. MRI examinations benefit from administering approximately 1 l of water in the 60 min prior to the exam. The imaging protocol should include: T1-weighted fat-suppressed spoiled gradient echo (SGE) imaging before

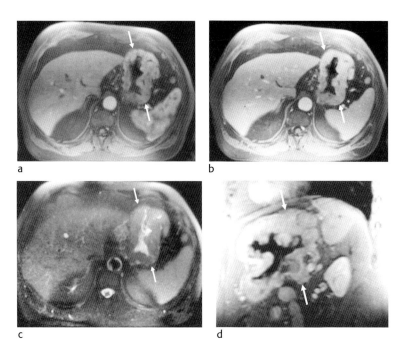

Figure 7.30a–d. Gastric cancer: MR features. Immediate postgadolinium (a) and 90-second-delayed
(b) axial T1-weighted fat-suppressed MR images show diffuse thickening of the gastric body with
increased mural enhancement. (c) T2-weighted fat-suppressed contrast-enhanced image confirms
the mural thickening as well as a hepatic cyst. (d) Sagittal T1-weighted fat-suppressed image shows
inhomogeneous intensity of the gastric wall. Arrows: gastric tumor.

and after the intravenous administration of gadolinium; unenhanced T1-weighted
SGE imaging; and T2-weighted single-shot echo-train spin-echo imaging. Gastric
mucosa enhances more intensely than other bowel mucosa after intravenous gadolinium injection.

On T1-weighted sequences, gastric adenocarcinoma is isointense to normal
stomach and may manifest only with mural thickening. On T2-weighted images,
gastric tumors are slightly higher in signal intensity than adjacent normal stomach.
It is important that there is adequate gastric distention. It is important to note that
collapsed normal gastric wall enhances identically to the remainder of the wall on
early and late postgadolinium images, as opposed to tumors which show more heterogeneous enhancement that may be increased or decreased relative to normal
gastric wall on early, late, or both sets of images.

Diffusely infiltrative carcinoma (linitis plastica) tends to have lower signal
intensity than normal adjacent stomach on T2-weighted images because of its

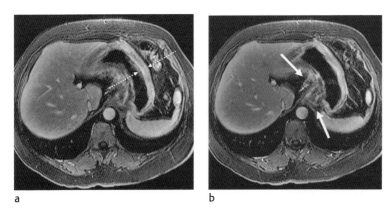

a   b

Figure 7.31a,b. Linitis plastica: MR features. T1-weighted, gadolinium-enhanced axial MR images show mural thickening of the stomach with increased enhancement (discontinuous arrows) and invasion of the gastrohepatic ligament (solid arrows).

desmoplastic nature. These tumors enhance only modestly after intravenous contrast whereas other histologic types of gastric tumors enhance more robustly with intravenous gadolinium. Fat-suppressed, gadolinium-enhanced SGE imaging assists the identification of transmural spread of tumor including peritoneal disease and tumor involvement of lymph nodes. Metastases enhance robustly against a background of low-signal-intensity fat.

T staging

In addition to conventional MRI with surface coils, endoluminal MRI with probes has shown some promise in T staging. Initial studies that reported an accuracy of 88% [109] and 81% [103] have not been duplicated. Problems include the small size of the serosa, and the lack of serosa in certain parts of the cardia region. Inflammatory reaction can also lead to overstaging.

In-vitro studies have shown that MRI has great promise in the depiction of gastric neoplasms that correlate well with histopathologic staging. Sato *et al.* [110] found that all T1-weighted, T2-weighted, and STIR (short tau inversion recovery) images consistently depicted the normal gastric wall as consisting of six layers and that MRI was 100% accurate in staging the depth of tumor invasion. In another in-vitro study, Palmowski *et al.* [106] found that infiltration of the subserosal and serosal layers was not accurately depicted, with overstaging of T2 tumors and only 50% accuracy in differentiating T2 from T3 tumors.

Endoluminal radiofrequency (RF) coils for MRI improve image quality and spatial resolution when compared to conventional MRI. A major problem with endoluminal RF coils is placement close to the region of interest and depth of visu-alization. A foldable and self-expanding loop coil design is used which enhances spatial resolution and depth of visualization. Using endoluminal MRI, Heye *et al.* [105] showed an overall accuracy for T staging of 75% with a sensitivity for detect-ing serosal involvement of 80% and a specificity of 89%.

N staging

In the detection of adenopathy, both CT and MRI depend upon lymph node size, number, and morphology. Tumor in normal sized nodes will remain undetected and enlarged lymph nodes due to infection or inflammation will errone-ously be considered positive, resulting in tumor understaging and overstaging, respectively.

To improve the accuracy of lymph node staging, Tatsumi and coworkers [111] have evaluated ferumoxtran-10, a lymphotropic contrast agent for MRI. In nor-mal lymph nodes, dark signal intensity is observed because of the diffuse uptake of contrast by macrophages resident in the lymph nodes which phagocytose the iron oxide particles of ferumoxtran-10. The number of phagocytic macrophages is decreased in nodes involved by tumor. In that study, three enhancement pat-terns were observed in lymph nodes: (A) lymph nodes with overall dark signal intensity due to diffuse iron uptake; (B) lymph nodes with partial high signal intensity due to partial uptake; (C) no blackening of nodes due to absent iron uptake. Patterns B and C were defined as lymph nodes positive for metastatic disease. The sensitivity, specificity, positive predictive value, negative predictive value, and overall predictive accuracy of post-contrast MRI were 100%, 92.6%, 85.5%, 100%, and 94.8%, respectively. These parameters for predictive accuracy were superior to CT and EUS. Nodes in the retroperitoneal and para-aortic regions were more readily identified and diagnosed on MRI than those in the perigastric region.

M staging

Magnetic resonance imaging is a superb means for detecting liver metastases and in many studies this imaging modality has proven slightly better than MDCT in lesion detection and characterization. MRI has also proven useful in the depic-tion of peritoneal metastases. Overall the accuracy of MRI in detecting metastatic disease at all sites is not significantly better than MDCT and as a consequence is primarily used as a problem-solving tool in patients with gastric cancer, rather than the initial staging examination [103, 104].

Assessing tumor response to therapy

In a study performed by Lee and others [112] CT volumetry was useful in predicting pathologic response following neoadjuvant chemotherapy in patients with resectable AGC. It compared volume changes of the primary gastric tumor and index lymph node. If the percentage volume reduction rate obtained at 8 weeks after neoadjuvant chemotherapy exceeds 35.6%, patients could be categorized as pathologic responders with 100% accuracy and 58.8% specificity.

Most medical centers and clinical trials use the RECIST criteria for measuring tumor response to therapy.

Recurrent gastric cancer

Earlier diagnosis of gastric cancer and more successful surgery together have greatly increased the number of patients requiring follow-up. There are three major reasons to follow up patients with gastric cancer: to detect problems associated with the operation, to collect outcomes data, and to detect recurrent disease. The active investigation of patients in order to detect recurrences at an earlier and asymptomatic stage is performed in the hope that this will lead to improved outcomes. The evidence for this is weak. While many national bodies and cancer organizations have offered guidelines for the follow-up of colon, breast, and lung cancers, guidelines for gastric cancer are notable by their absence. Indeed the Japanese Gastric Cancer Association guidelines, which are proscriptive in the diagnosis and surgical treatment of gastric cancer, offer no guidance for follow-up [110, 111, 112, 113, 114, 115, 116, 117, 118, 119, 120, 121, 122, 123].

Gastric cancer has four major patters of recurrence: local recurrence in the gastric bed or regional lymph nodes; peritoneal dissemination; liver metastases; and distant metastases. Risk factors for recurrent tumor include greater stage of the disease, undifferentiated tumor type, and proximal tumors [110, 111, 112, 113, 114, 115, 116, 117, 118, 119, 120, 121, 122, 123].

In the West, recurrences tend to be local. In one series, distant metastases were found in 26% but local recurrence was present in 88% of patients [115]. In an Italian series, 45% suffered local recurrence, 27% had hepatic metastases, 36% showed peritoneal disease, and 9% had distant metastases [116]. In the East, the pattern is different with fewer local recurrences. In a series from Japan [117], recurrence was local in 22%, peritoneal in 43%, hepatic in 33%, distant in 21%, and 25% had recurrences at multiple sites. In a large Korean series, 23% had local recurrence, 40% had peritoneal recurrence, 18% had hepatic metastases, and 19% had distant metastases [89].

The lower local recurrence rate in the East appears to be related to the routine performance of D2 lymphadenectomies, as use of this technique in the West leads to comparable low local recurrence rates.

It appears that over two-thirds of recurrences occur within the first 3 years and that fewer than 10% occur after 5 years [120]. In EGC, the majority (62%) of recurrences are detected at less than 2 years and fewer than 10% occur after 5 years [89]. Adjuvant treatment after gastrectomy may also alter patterns of recurrence. MacDonald *et al.* [121], in an adjuvant chemoradiation study, reported that adjuvant treatment reduced the proportion of patients recorded as having local and regional recurrences as the first site of relapse from 29% and 72% respectively in the surgery-alone group to 19% and 65% in the patients who also had chemoradiation.

Specific pathologic features of the resected tumor can provide insights into the likely pathways of recurrence, allowing follow-up plans to be tailored to the individual patient. In patients with T1, T2, N0 neoplasms with histologic evidence of venous capillary infiltration, recurrence is invariably by hepatic metastases. Although bone metastases are relatively uncommon, in poorly differentiated carcinomas or SRCs with very extensive nodal involvement, they are more likely, and some may respond to chemotherapy [122].

Even after potentially curative gastrectomy, tumor recurs in nearly 70% of patients, usually within 2 years. Tumor recurrence and survival are strongly dependent upon tumor stage and the extent of surgical resection. Recurrent tumor following radical resection is caused by progressive development of micrometastases, with 40%–50% locoregional recurrence, 34%–54 % involving the peritoneum, and 54%–76% involving distant sites [70]. When recurrence occurs, any treatments with a curative intent are usually futile. Recently however, secondary total gastrectomy has been attempted if the local recurrence is confined to the stomach and long-term survival is improved significantly. The importance of early detection of locoregional recurrence after gastrectomy must be emphasized.

Endoscopy, double-contrast barium studies, and MDCT have been used to detect recurrent tumors of the remnant stomach. Surgical alterations of the anatomy usually limit the value of these tests, and surgical plication defects in particular are a potential source of erroneous interpretation of local recurrence. In one study it was found that malignant wall thickening in the postoperative stomach is characterized by a thicker wall (0.24 mm), enhancement equal to or greater than normal mucosa, perigastric infiltration apart from the metallic suture material, heterogeneous mural enhancement, obliteration of mural stratification, lymphadenopathy, and adjacent bowel wall thickening [117].

Tumor recurrence has a poor prognosis, however early recognition is helpful because the patient with minimal adenopathy or small recurrent masses may show an improved response to chemotherapy or radiation therapy.

MDCT is the primary imaging test for evaluating suspected recurrences but often cannot differentiate treatment-induced morphologic changes from tumor recurrence. Recurrence at the gastric stump or anastomosis manifests as nonspecific mural thickening. Inadequate distention, surgical plication defects, bowel adhesions, and gastritis are potential sources of erroneous interpretation. Since FDG uptake is elevated in tumor and low in scar tissue, PET-CT can better characterize equivocal CT findings that are suggestive of tumor recurrence. FDG-PET however may be limited by tumor type. PET-CT is also useful in following the response of the primary gastric neoplasm to neoadjuvant chemotherapy (Figure 7.28).

Gastric lymphoma

Introduction

Gastric lymphoma includes both primary gastric lymphoma and systemic lymphoma with secondary gastric involvement. The GI tract is the most common extranodal site of involvement by systemic lymphoma and more than 50% of patients with non-Hodgkin lymphoma have GI tract involvement. The stomach is the most common GI site followed by the small intestine, the ileocecal region, and colon. Primary gastric lymphomas are those tumors without systemic involvement until very late in the disease. Confirmatory criteria for primary gastric lymphoma include: no palpable adenopathy, normal peripheral blood smear and bone marrow examination, no mediastinal adenopathy, lymphoma limited to the stomach, and no hepatic or splenic involvement except by direct extension [124, 125, 126, 127, 128].

The commonest lymphomas encountered in the stomach are extranodal marginal zone B cell lymphoma of mucosa-associated lymphoid tissue (MALT) type and diffuse B cell lymphomas. The stomach may also be infiltrated in up to 25% of nodal type of lymphomas [124, 125, 126, 127, 128].

MALT lymphoma is a distinctive type of lymphoma that manifests as localized disease and generally has a favorable prognosis. The gastric mucosa normally does not contain lymphatic tissue, and MALT lymphoma is associated with follicular gastritis caused by *H. pylori*. Low-grade MALT lymphoma shows a diffuse infiltrate of small centrocyte-like cells that may invade the epithelial lining of glands or crypts and form lymphoepithelial lesions. In high-grade MALT lymphoma, large lymphoid cells transform from low-grade MALT lymphoma to form confluent clusters or sheets with or without areas of a low-grade component.

Several staging systems (Table 7.2 and Figure 7.32) have been proposed for classifying gastric lymphoma. These include the Ann Arbor, Musshoff, and Blackledge systems. The Ann Arbor system is the most widely used but does not distinguish regional from extra-regional nodal involvement whereas the Musshoff system does make this distinction. The Blackledge system includes an additional stage for locally advanced disease, serosal involvement, perforation, or adherence or involvement of adjacent structures. It lacks a Stage III designating nodal involvement on both sides of the diaphragm [124, 125, 126, 127, 128].

Accurate staging is an important prognostic factor, as are an association with human immunodeficiency virus (HIV), clinical presentation with acute abdomen, tumor size, tumor histology, and level of tumor invasion (Table 7.3).

Patterns of tumor spread

The stomach is most commonly involved by MALT lymphoma followed by the colorectum and small bowel. MALT lymphoma has also been reported in Barrett

Table 7.2. Staging systems for gastric lymphoma

Feature	Ann Arbor	Musshoff	Blackledge	5YS[1]
Confined to GI tract	IE	IE	I	80
Nodal involvement (infradiaphragmatic)	IIE			40
Regional nodes		IIE1	II1	50
Extra-regional nodes		IIE2	II2	35
Serosal involvement+adjacent structures			IIE	15
Nodal involvement (infra- and supradiaphragmatic)	IIIE	IIIE		30
Non-GI extranodal involvement	IVE	IVE	IV	5

[1] 5YS, 5-year survival.

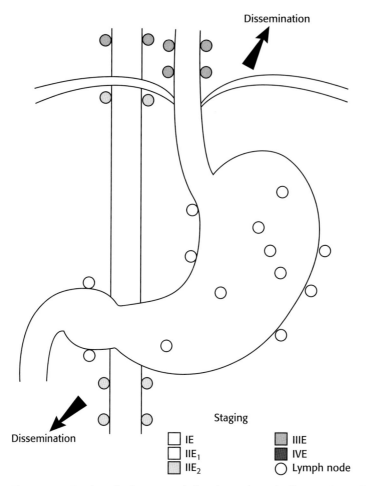

Dissemination

Dissemination

Staging

IE

IIE₁

IIE₂

IIIE

IVE

○ Lymph node

Figure 7.32. Staging of primary gastric lymphoma (Musshoff system). Staging of primary gastric lymphoma is analogous to staging of other extranodal lymphomas; E denotes extranodal. Stage IE involves only the stomach. Stage IIE involves infradiaphragmatic nodes; IIE1 designates regional (contiguous) nodes, and IIE2 indicates extraregional nodes. Stage IIIE involves supradiaphragmatic nodes as well, and stage IV is disseminated disease. From Luk GD. Tumors of the stomach. In Feldman M, Scharschmidt BF, and Sleisenger MH eds., *Gastrointestinal and Liver Disease*, 6th edn. Philadelphia, PA: WB Saunders, 1998; pp. 733–60, Figure 44–16, p. 751.

esophagus and in the gallbladder. In cases of multifocal involvement, gene rearrangement studies suggest that the separate tumors are derived from a single clone of cells which may develop into closely related populations of subclones. In disseminated, Stage IV gastric lymphoma the most common sites of spread are: lymph nodes beneath the diaphragm (46%); bone marrow (43%); other GI

Table 7.3. Prognostic features of gastric lymphoma

Good prognosis
Tumor smaller than 10 cm in diameter
Submucosal involvement only
Diffuse or large-cell histology
MALT features
Musshoff stage IE or IIE1
Resectable for cure

Poor prognosis
Association with HIV
Presentation with acute abdomen
Lesser curvature tumors
Tumors larger than 10 cm in diameter
Immunoblastic histology
T cell tumors
Tumor with aneuploidy
Later Musshoff stage than IIE2

tract sites (22%); liver (19%); head and neck (8%); lymph nodes above the diaphragm (5%); Waldeyer's ring (5%); spleen (5%); respiratory tract (3%); and central nervous system (3%) [124, 125, 126, 127, 128].

Endoscopic ultrasound

Endoscopic US (Figures 7.33 and 7.34) has proven to be very useful in the diagnosis and staging of gastric lymphomas. When combined with endoscopy and biopsy, the diagnostic accuracy can approach 100% and staging accuracy is about 80%, obviating the need for staging laparotomy in most patients. EUS can provide information concerning the depth of tumor invasion and abnormal local lymph nodes [129].

Endoscopic US is the most accurate method for staging localized MALT lymphoma. As in patients with gastric adenocarcinoma, EUS can depict the histologic layers of the gastric wall and identify layers that are thickened due to tumor involvement. EUS-guided fine-needle aspiration biopsy can also be used to obtain cytologic and histologic material when standard endoscopic biopsies are insufficient. Staging with EUS has also been shown to accurately predict response to antibiotic therapy. EUS features of gastric lymphoma include: localized

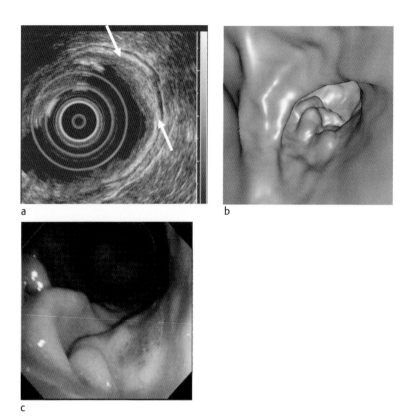

a   b

c

Figure 7.33a–c. MALT lymphoma: imaging features. (a) EUS shows mural thickening of the gastric mucosa (arrows). (b) VG demonstrates focal thickening of the rugal folds of the stomach. (c) Upper GI endoscopy shows a raised lesion with mucosal erythema.

non-homogeneous polypoid matrix; local or diffuse hypoechoic infiltration; mural thickening with superficial ulcerations; and multiple hypoechoic mass lesions [130, 131].

Computed tomography

MALT lymphoma

CT is useful in differentiating high-grade from low-grade MALT lymphomas. Most low-grade lymphomas show superficial spreading lesions with mucosal nodularity, shallow ulcer, and minimal fold thickening. Most high-grade lymphomas show mass-forming lesions or severe fold thickening [131, 132].

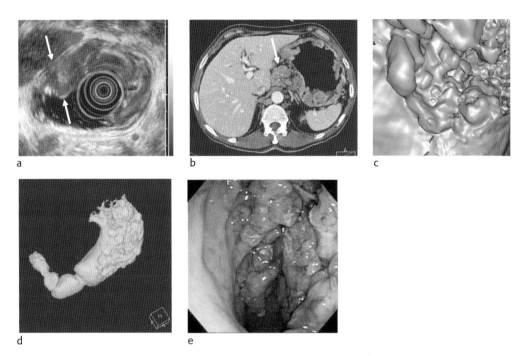

Figure 7.34a–e. Diffuse gastric lymphoma. (a) EUS shows marked gastric wall thickening (arrows). (b) Wall thickening is also demonstrated on this CT scan, which also shows adenopathy in the gastrohepatic ligament (arrow). VG (c), shaded surface display (d), and upper GI endoscopy (e) images show thickened rugal folds.

In one series [132], CT was normal in 28% of patients with low-grade lymphoma whereas all patients with high-grade lymphoma showed imaging abnormalities. The mural thickening in low-grade lymphoma had a mean of 0.8 cm compared to a mean of 2.5 cm in patients with high-grade lymphoma. Abdominal adenopathy was observed in 14% of patients with low-grade lymphoma but in 75% of patients with high-grade lymphoma.

In another study [133], CT showed different features for the two types of lymphoma. CT was abnormal in 100% of patients with high-grade lymphoma and in only 51% of patients with low-grade lymphoma. Gastric wall thickening was also more diffuse (48% vs 8%) and severe (71% vs 14%) than in the low-grade group. Lymphadenopathy was visualized in 67% of the high-grade group and only in 5% of the low-grade group. Gastric ulcers were identified on CT in 57% of the high-grade group and in only 5% of the low-grade group [133].

Gastric wall thickening is the leading CT finding in non-Hodgkin lymphoma (Figure 7.35). Mural thickness is generally greater than 1 cm and the mean thickness ranges from 2.9 to 5 cm. Thickening affects the wall of the entire stomach in 50% of cases. Otherwise the areas of predominant involvement are the antrum, body, and fundus. Lesions in the proximal part of the stomach are often of the segmental form whereas antral involvement is of the diffuse form. Mural thickening typically involves more than half the circumference of the gastric lumen and more than one region of the stomach is involved. These findings typify the submucosal spread of gastric lymphoma [134, 135, 136, 137, 138].

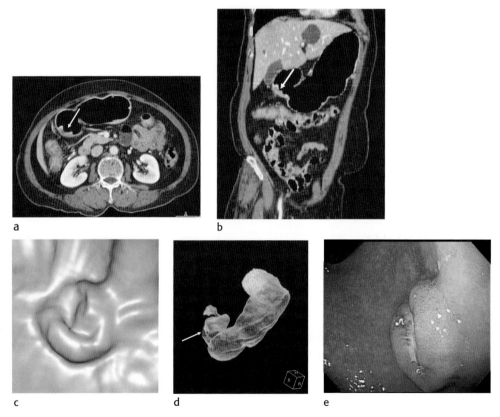

a   b   c   d   e

Figure 7.35a–e. Polypoid gastric lymphoma: imaging features. Axial (a) and coronal (b) CT scans show focal mural thickening in the region of the gastric antrum (arrows). This lesion is also depicted on the VG (c), shaded surface display (d), and upper GI endoscopy (e) images.

In gastric lymphoma, the mural thickening usually is homogeneous but may be inhomogeneous due to the presence of necrosis, hemorrhage, submucosal edema, or infarction. The outer gastric margin is usually smooth or lobulated whereas the inner gastric wall is frequently irregular in contour representing distortion of the thickened gastric rugae [134, 135, 136, 137, 138].

On CT, gastric lymphoma may be indistinguishable from adenocarcinomas. Features that favor gastric lymphoma over adenocarcinoma include: marked gastric wall thickening, more than one lesion, infrequent gastric outlet obstruction, and adenopathy that extends below the level of the renal hila [134, 135, 136, 137, 138].

In patients with known or suspected gastric lymphoma, 2D MPR and VG may allow both depiction of a gastric lesion and staging of generalized lymphoma in the abdomen [134]. Because the most frequent finding in both gastric lymphoma and gastric MALT lymphoma is mural thickening, careful attention to technique is needed. VG and 2D MPR provide clear visualization of the gross morphology of gastric lymphoma, including changes in the dimensions of the gastric lumen, the gastric wall, and perigastric adenopathy. VG affords better evaluation of the mucosal changes. VG can show mucosal nodularity, a shallow or deep ulcer, single or multiple masses, rugal thickening, and enlarged areae gastricae. VG and 2D MPR may permit early diagnosis of disease progression in patients undergoing therapy and follow-up for low-grade MALT lymphoma. EUS is more accurate for local tumor staging. In patients with MALT lymphoma it helps to determine the horizontal extent of the tumor, the depth of mural invasion, and the invasion of perigastric lymph nodes. Tumor regression is recognized as normalization of wall thickness at EUS [134].

Magnetic resonance imaging

As with adenocarcinoma of the stomach, MRI has a limited role in the evaluation of patients with gastric lymphoma. Mural thickening is the hallmark of gastric lymphoma on MRI. Non-Hodgkin lymphoma preserves gastric distensibility. The thickened gastric wall typically shows homogeneous signal intensity (Figure 7.36) and moderate contrast enhancement. Diffuse gastric wall thickening is best seen on single-shot echo-train spin-echo and gadolinium-enhanced fat-suppressed SGE images. Tumor-containing lymph nodes can also be depicted with these imaging sequences [129].

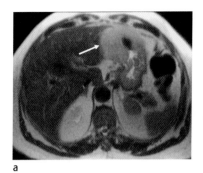
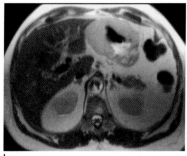

a   b

Figure 7.36a,b. Gastric lymphoma: MR features. Axial images (a) and (b) show homogeneous mural thickening (arrow) of the angulus and proximal antrum of the stomach.

Gastrointestinal stromal tumors

Introduction

Gastrointestinal stromal tumors (GISTs) constitute the majority of all GI mesenchymal tumors. Formerly, they were classified as leiomyomas and leiomyosarcomas; GISTs are now recognized as a distinct class of mesenchymal tumors that are separate from true smooth muscle tumors of the GI tract. They have a different etiology, immunohistology, and clinical course.

Gastrointestinal stromal tumors arise within the muscularis propria of the GI wall and can occur anywhere in the GI tract from the esophagus to the rectum, but arise most frequently in the stomach (60%), followed by the small intestine (20%–30%), the colon, rectum, and esophagus. They may also occur primarily in the omentum, mesentery, retroperitoneum, gallbladder or bladder. GISTs are submucosal in origin with a predilection for extraluminal development. They are highly vascular neoplasms with a tendency to undergo necrosis, which explains their heterogeneous appearance [139, 140, 141, 142, 143, 144, 145, 146, 147, 148].

These tumors express the c-kit proto-oncogene protein, a cell membrane receptor with tyrosine kinase activity. A mutation in the c-kit proto-oncogene results in activation of the KIT receptor tyrosine kinase, which leads to unchecked cell growth and resistance to apoptosis. The development of a KIT tyrosine kinase inhibitor, imatinib mesylate (Gleevec), has made it vital to distinguish GISTs from other mesenchymal tumors of the GI tract [139, 140, 141, 142, 143, 144, 145, 146, 147, 148].

Gastrointestinal stromal tumors are rare in patients younger than 40 years, occurring predominantly in middle-aged patients. Most patients with GIST are symptomatic and bleeding due to mucosal ulceration, which is the most common symptom [139, 140, 141, 142, 143, 144, 145, 146, 147, 148].

Surgery remains the mainstay of treatment in patients with localized GISTs. The principal surgery is R0 resection of the tumor. Tumor rupture or R1 resection of the primary tumor has a negative impact on disease-free survival. Lower local recurrence rates occur with segmental resection of the stomach compared to wedge resection [143].

The new trend in cancer therapy is a treatment directed at specific, frequently occurring molecular alterations in signaling pathways of cancer cells. Mutations in c-kit receptors occur in 80%–85% of GISTs so a targeted treatment by a tyrosine kinase inhibitor of the kit receptor such as imatinib mesylate shows effectiveness against primary and metastatic tumors [145].

Pathologic features and risk stratification

Criteria for distinguishing malignant from benign GISTs have been sought, analyzed, and debated for years. Accurate risk stratification of gastric GISTs is becoming increasingly important because of emerging adjuvant systemic treatments. All GISTs are considered to have some malignant potential. Gastric GISTs have a better prognosis than non-gastric tumors of the same size and mitotic count and serosal invasion. Clearly tumor rupture confers increased risk. The National Institutes of Health (NIH) has delineated risk factors and their relationship to the clinical aggressiveness of the tumor. Patients considered at very low risk have a tumor size of < 2 cm and a mitotic count of < 5 per 50 high power fields (HPFs). Low-risk patients have a tumor size of 2–5 cm, and mitotic count of < 5 per 50 HPFs. Those patients with intermediate risk have tumors > 5 cm in size and a mitotic count of 6–10 per 50 HPFs or a tumor size of 5–10 cm with a mitotic count of < 5 per 50 HPF. High-risk patients have tumors > 5 cm in size with a mitotic count of > 5 per 50 HPF, tumor size > 10 cm with any mitotic rate, or tumors of any size with a mitotic count > 10 per 50 HPF [144, 145, 146].

Imaging features

Unlike most GI epithelial tumors, the majority of GISTs (76%) are exophytic in growth, so that obstruction is uncommon even in the setting of very large tumors. These tumors may undergo extensive necrosis and fistula formation resulting in the formation of a cavity within the mass and bleeding. GISTs which have a fistulous

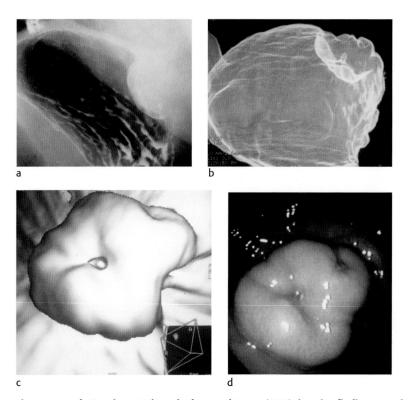

Figure 7.37a–d. Gastric gastrointestinal stromal tumor (GIST): imaging findings. An ulcerated submucosal tumor is identified along the greater curvature aspect of the stomach on an upper GI series (a) and shaded surface display (b) CT image. Note the nice correlation between the VG (c) and upper GI endoscopy (d) images.

tract to the gut may show an air–fluid level. Orally administered positive contrast material may also be seen within the mass. After the intravenous administration of contrast material, large tumors demonstrate heterogeneous enhancement, while smaller tumors may present homogeneous enhancement [149, 150, 151, 152, 153, 154, 155, 156, 157, 158, 159, 160, 161, 162, 163, 164, 165].

The presence of focal areas of low attenuation in GIST tumors is a nonspecific finding that can be seen in a variety of pathologic conditions such as hypocellular tumor, hemorrhage, necrosis, cystic degeneration, and fluid in an ulcer. Accordingly these low-density areas in small GISTs are not predictors of malignant potential [155].

Multidetector CT (MDCT) (Figures 7.37, 7.38, 7.39, 7.40, 7.41, 7.42) has proven to be the most useful means of detecting patients with GISTs. These lesions are often found incidentally. Small tumors manifest as intramural masses. As the tumor

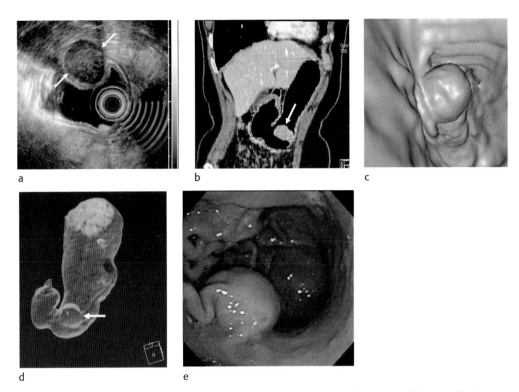

Figure 7.38a–e. Gastric GIST: imaging findings. (a) EUS image shows a well marginated intramural mass (arrows) with homogeneous echo architecture. (b) Corresponding coronal MPR image shows that this endophytic lesion (arrow) originates from the greater curvature of the gastric angulus. VG (c), shaded surface display (d), and upper GI endoscopy (e) images show this smooth marginated neoplasm (arrow).

grows, the overlying mucosa can ulcerate. Imaging features that suggest malignancy include a large tumor size, an exophytic mass, and a mass containing areas of central necrosis or calcification. When tumors are large and exophytic, it may be difficult to identify the organ of origin. It is unusual to find adenopathy in patients with GISTs. CT can show the spectrum of findings in patients with Carney's triad, a rare syndrome in which patients develop GISTs, pulmonary chondromas, and extra-adrenal paragangliomas (Figure 7.43).

Virtual gastroscopy can be helpful in better characterizing the mass and determining its origin. 2D MPR is very useful in evaluating exophytic growth patterns, lymphadenopathy, and distant-organ metastases. Most tumors appear as well-defined submucosal masses. VG affords nice depiction of smooth, well-defined masses with a central ulcer, at right angles or slightly obtuse angles with the adjacent wall, and the bridging folds at the margin of the mass. Transparency rendering

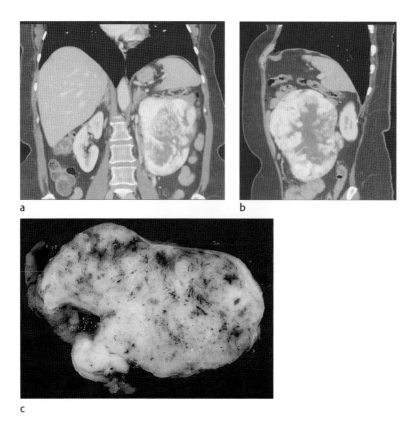

a   b

c

Figure 7.39a–c. Hypervascular exophytic gastric GIST: CT features. Coronal (a) and sagittal (b) MPR images show a strikingly vascular neoplasm. (c) Pathologic correlation.

provides a useful preoperative map and global orientation of the submucosal mass in the stomach, which is useful for the surgeon. EUS can demonstrate the layer of origin of the submucosal tumor [65].

Kim *et al.* [153] reported that the presence of an ulcer, mesenteric fat infiltration, direct organ invasion, and metastases are more frequently seen in patients with a high mitotic rate. In the same report, no CT feature other than size was found to have predictive value with respect to malignant gastric GISTs.

Imaging follow-up of GISTs

With the new generation of molecular target agents such as imatinib mesylate, it appears that conventional objective response criteria such as lesion size are

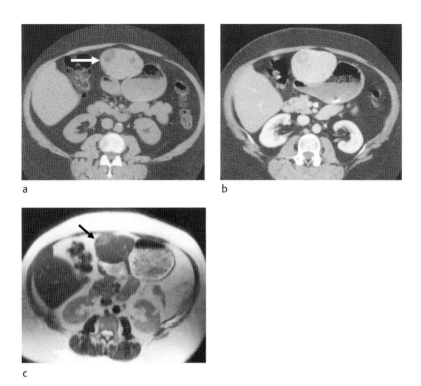

a   b

c

Figure 7.40a–c. GIST: MR-CT correlation. (a) Pre- and (b) post-contrast-enhanced CT scans show a well marginated, slightly inhomogeneous, enhancing mass (arrow) arising from the lesser curvature aspect of the stomach. (c) MR fat-suppressed T2-weighted image shows similar features.

no longer sufficient to assess tumor response to therapy. The difference in metabolic activity after even a single dose of imatinib mesylate can be dramatic on FDG-PET while little or no change may be seen on the corresponding CT scan [166, 167].

In a pilot study Holdsworth *et al.* [167] compared the CT bidirectional measurements and FDG-PET standard uptake value (SUV) in determining response to imatinib mesylate treatment. The best metrics were the optimized PET SUV threshold of 3.4 at 1 month.

Lassau *et al.* [168] reported that contrast-enhanced Doppler sonography allows early and accurate evaluation of the efficacy of imatinib. Decreased contrast uptake observed on days 7 and 17 after the beginning of treatment was correlated with a good response at 2 months.

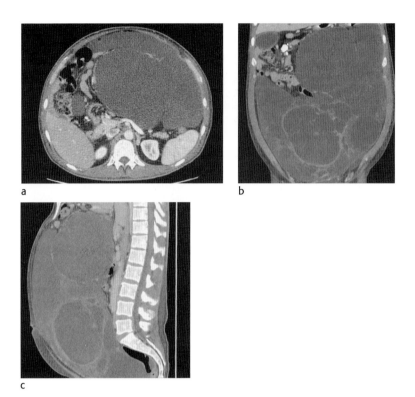

Figure 7.41a–c. Cystic exophytic gastric GIST with peritoneal dissemination: CT findings. Axial (a), coronal (b), and sagittal (c) scans show a large, cystic septated mass that raises suspicion of carcinomatosis due to a mucinous ovarian or GI tract malignancy. Pathologically this proved to be a large cystic GIST tumor.

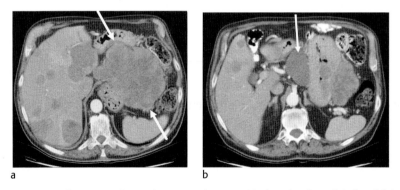

Figure 7.42a,b. Metastatic gastric GIST: CT features. (a) There is a large lobulated, inhomogeneous mass (arrows) arising along the greater curvature aspect of the stomach. Note the multiple low-density hepatic metastases. (b) Scan obtained caudal to (a) shows mural thickening of the stomach and a cystic metastasis (arrow) in the gastrohepatic ligament.

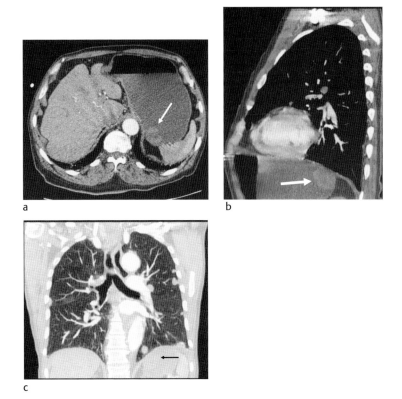

Figure 7.43a–c. Carney's triad: CT features. This is a rare syndrome in which GISTs, pulmonary chondromas, and extra-adrenal paragangliomas develop in the same patient. Axial (a) and sagittal (b) CT images show a mass (arrows) in the posterior aspect of the stomach. (c) Coronal MPR image displayed at lung windows shows the mass (arrow) and multiple pulmonary chondromas.

Vanel and coworkers [169] have reported that in patients with hepatic and peritoneal metastases, a decrease in density (Figure 7.44) and contrast enhancement of these lesions with overall stable size collectively signifies a good response to therapy. Following contrast administration, marked enhancement is seen peripherally, with a less vascular center explaining the central necrosis often seen. The enhancement begins on the arterial phase in the periphery, with progressive centripetal opacification. Changes in internal tumor structure with near fluid level of hepatic metastases with residual masses may indicate a good response. Accordingly, size criteria should not be the sole indication of treatment response. A solid nodule appearing within a cystic residual mass indicates early tumor recurrence [167, 168, 169, 170, 171, 172, 173, 174, 175, 176].

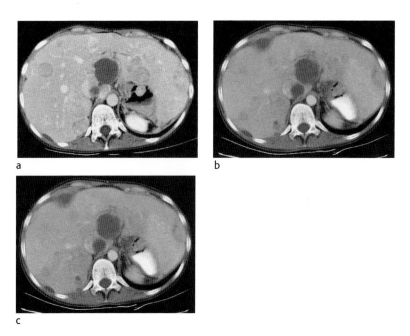

Figure 7.44a–c. CT assessment of tumor response to imatinib mesylate in a patient with metastatic gastric GIST. (a) Pre-therapy axial scan shows solid and cystic metastases. These metastases become relatively cystic (b) and (c) following therapy.

Mabille *et al.* [177] also reported that the development of peripheral mural thickening or enhancing nodules within cystic-like metastatic lesions, even without any change in size, represents tumor progression.

Carcinoid tumors

Introduction

Carcinoid tumors represent a group of well-differentiated tumors originating from the diffuse endocrine system outside the pancreas and thyroid. Carcinoids most often occur in the gut (66.9%) followed by the tracheobronchial system (24.5%). Gastric carcinoids account for 8.7% of all GI carcinoids and 1.8% of gastric malignancies.

Gastric carcinoid tumors are more common in women than men [178, 179, 180, 181].

In the GI tract, gastric carcinoids originate from the endocrine cells that populate the mucosa and submucosa. The majority are enterochromaffin-like cells (ECL

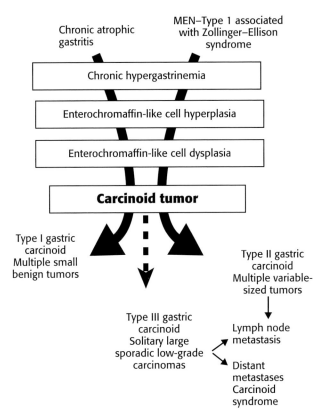

Chronic atrophic
gastritis

MEN–Type 1 associated
with Zollinger–Ellison
syndrome

Chronic hypergastrinemia

Enterochromaffin-like cell hyperplasia

Enterochromaffin-like cell dysplasia

Carcinoid tumor

Type I gastric
carcinoid
Multiple small
benign tumors

Type II gastric
carcinoid
Multiple variable-
sized tumors

Type III gastric
carcinoid
Solitary large
sporadic low-grade
carcinomas

Lymph node
metastasis

Distant
metastases
Carcinoid
syndrome

Figure 7.45. Drawing shows pathophysiologic schema for development of different types of gastric carcinoid tumors. Type I carcinoid tumors are small benign tumors, arising in the setting of chronic atrophic gastritis and chronic hypergastrinemia. Type II tumors can be large and polypoid; arise in patients with multiple endocrine neoplasia-type I and Zollinger–Ellison syndrome; and are prone to nodal metastasis. Type III tumors, which are not associated with the hypergastrinemic state, are large, sporadic, solitary tumors that are prone to nodal and hepatic metastases, as well as to carcinoid syndrome. From Binstock AJ, Johnson CD, Stephens DH et al. Carcinoid tumors of the stomach: a clinical and radiographic study. AJR Am J Roentgenol 176 (2001), 947–51, Figure 5, p. 950.

cells) that arise from oxyntic mucosa in the gastric body and fundus. Because of their neuroendocrine origin, carcinoids are characterized by the secretion of a variety of neuropeptides and amines that can lead to clinical symptoms and the carcinoid syndrome. The majority of gastroduodenal carcinoids, however, are indolent and asymptomatic [178, 179, 180, 181].

Gastric carcinoids are divided into three subtypes (Figure 7.45), which include an assessment of comorbid conditions and the presence of ECL hyperplasia. ECL cells have been implicated in the pathogenesis of poorly differentiated and highly malignant neuroendocrine carcinoma of the stomach [182, 183, 184].

Type I ECL cells are the most common type, representing 74% of gastric endocrine tumors. They occur most commonly in women (F:M ratio of 2.5) with a mean age of 63 years. Patients do not have symptoms directly related to the tumors. These lesions are usually encountered during endoscopy performed for dyspepsia, anemia that may be due to chronic atrophic gastritis, or other reasons. Achlorhydria and less commonly pernicious anemia may be present. Hypergastrinemia or evidence of antral G-cell hyperplasia is usually observed. Type I gastric carcinoid is generally considered a benign disease with only rare (2%) nodal and liver metastases. These patients can be treated conservatively with endoscopic surveillance and local treatment for tumors ≤ 1 cm and partial gastric resection for tumors > 1 cm. Radiographic studies may underestimate the number of gastric carcinoid tumors [182, 183, 184].

Type II gastric ECL-cell carcinoids are the least common type, accounting for 6% of gastric endocrine neoplasms, and occur at a mean age of 50 years with no gender predilection. These tumors are seen in association with the hypergastrinemic state of Zollinger–Ellison syndrome associated with multiple endocrine neoplasia type 1 (MEN-1). Approximately 30% of patients with MEN-1 will have gastric carcinoid tumors. Clinically, elevated gastrin levels produce signs and symptoms of a hypertrophic, hypersecretory gastritis: abdominal pain or bleeding from multiple or recurrent peptic ulcers, diarrhea, and elevated levels of serum gastrin [185, 186].

Type II carcinoids can also arise from ECL cells in the setting of hyperplasia. These carcinoids tend to be multicentric and variable in size but are prone to developing local lymph node metastases. Carcinoid syndrome and tumor-related death are uncommon. On upper GI studies and CT, the appearance can be striking, with multiple masses associated with diffuse mural thickening of the stomach.

Type III tumors are sporadically occurring and represent about 20% of gastric carcinoids. There is a striking male predominance (80%). These tumors are highly proliferative and have an intense overexpression of the p53 proteins, which are encoded by a tumor suppressor gene that is thought to be responsible for apoptosis of damaged cells. These lesions are large solitary tumors that may show ulceration and are more likely to be invasive, with distant metastases. The presence of metastases is dependent on tumor size, with fewer than 10% of single tumors < 1 cm showing metastases and tumors > 3 cm often demonstrating metastases. Prognosis is poor, with only 20% of patients surviving 5 years. Carcinoid syndrome may be present in patients with liver metastases. Since type III tumors are aggressive, they should be treated with total gastrectomy and en-bloc removal of regional lymph nodes when liver metastases are absent. If liver metastases are present, systemic chemotherapy and antitumoral therapies are recommended [178, 179, 180, 181].

Nuclear medicine scans with radiolabeled somatostatin analogs can be used to identify the location of primary and metastatic carcinoid tumors and have been reported to have detection rates of 80%–90%.

Small localized tumors measuring < 2 cm that are confined to the submucosa without evidence of invasion of the muscularis propria or lymph node metastasis can be removed with minimally invasive endoscopic mucosal or submucosal resection. Close endoscopic follow-up is needed following these therapies [178, 179, 180, 181].

Tumors > 2 cm in size that are confined to the gastric wall should be surgically removed. Patients with multiple tiny gastric carcinoids should undergo close follow-up to see if these lesions are stable in size. In the setting of atrophic oxyntic gland gastritis with achlorhydria, these lesions often do not enlarge. Multiple lesions can be removed endoscopically. Patients with multiple large carcinoids may require total gastrectomy. The overall 5-year survival of patients with gastric carcinoids is 48.6% and for those with small intestinal tumors it is 55.4%. In the setting of regional lymph node metastases or distant metastases, prognosis is poor. Tumor size > 2 cm, invasion of the muscularis propria, poorly differentiated histology, and the presence of numerous mitotic figures on histology are findings associated with increased metastatic risk [178, 179, 180, 181].

Imaging features

Types I and II (Figure 7.46) ECL-cell carcinoids are multifocal, smoothly marginated, 1- to 2-cm mural masses located in the gastric body and fundus. They may appear as an enhancing mucosal or submucosal mass. Irrespective of cell type and biologic potential, larger carcinoids may have mucosal ulcerations on the surface of the mass. These ulcers are identified as focal, irregular collections of barium, contrast material or air on the surface of the mass. In the setting of Zollinger–Ellison syndrome and MEN-1 marked mural thickening of the stomach and innumerable nodular mucosal and mural masses may be present that show enhancement during the hepatic arterial phase. In patients with hypergastrinemia and suspected gastric carcinoids, gastric distention is important and scans should be obtained during the hepatic arterial and portal venous phases to maximize detection of the primary gastric lesions as well as liver metastases [182, 183, 184].

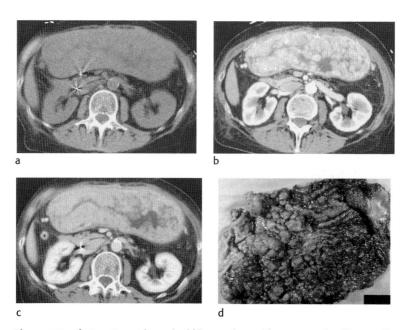

a   b

c   d

Figure 7.46a–d. Type II gastric carcinoid in a patient with MEN-1 and Zollinger–Ellison syndrome. (a) Non-contrast CT shows marked mural thickening of the stomach. (b) Scan obtained during the hepatic arterial phase shows innumerable enhancing nodules lining the thickened rugal folds. (c) Late portal venous phase scan shows the folds are homogeneous in attenuation. (d) Resected gastrectomy specimen reveals innumerable small nodules of carcinoid throughout the gastric mucosa. From Levy AD and Sobin LH. Gastrointestinal carcinoids: imaging features with clinicopathologic comparison. *Radiographics* 27 (2007), 237–57, Figure 4a–d, p. 243.

Type III ECL-cell carcinoids are solitary, large mural masses (Figure 7.47) in the body and fundus of the stomach which may be ulcerated. Because these lesions have a distinct malignant potential, imaging studies should be carried out for the presence of perigastric adenopathy and liver metastases [182, 183, 184].

Endoscopic US is useful in the evaluation of these tumors to determine the depth of invasion within the gastric wall and the presence or absence of associated adenopathy which would indicate malignancy. Sonographically, gastric carcinoids are hypoechoic and homogeneous with smooth margins. The majority are located within the submucosa but they can be seen invading the mucosa or the muscularis propria. The overall accuracy of EUS for determining depth of invasion is 90% and for local lymph node metastases it is 75% [182, 183, 184, 185, 186].

The differential diagnosis for types I and II ECL-cell gastric carcinoids includes disorders that cause multiple polypoid masses, such as multiple hyperplastic polyps, adenomatous and fundic gland polyps in familial adenomatous polyposis

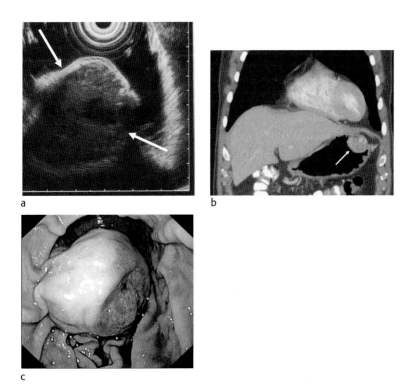

a

b

c

Figure 7.47a–c. Type III gastric carcinoid: imaging features. A well-marginated mass (arrows) is identified in the gastric fundus on EUS (a), coronal MPR-CT (b), and upper GI endoscopy (c) images.

syndrome, hamartomatous polyps in Peutz–Jeghers syndrome, juvenile polyposis, Cronkhite–Canada syndrome, and Cowden disease. Metastases and Kaposi sarcoma, gastric adenocarcinoma, lymphoma, and GIST are the major differential diagnostic considerations in patients with type III ECL-cell carcinoids [187,188].

Summary

Despite recent advances in the detection, staging, and therapy of gastric carcinoma, it remains a lethal disease. In the future, improvements in overall patient survival can only be achieved by tailored therapeutic strategies, which are based on individual histologic tumor type, tumor location, tumor stage at the time of presentation, consideration of established prognostic factors, and the physiologic status of the patient. Elucidation of the biochemical and genetic events that regulate and correlate with different stages of carcinogenesis will lead to the development of markers that can be employed diagnostically, prognostically, and therapeutically.

Innovations in novel molecular-based and biologic therapeutic agents such as an epidermal growth factor antagonist will be required to improve therapy-related outcomes and minimize treatment-related side-effects.

Because prognosis is so closely related to stage at the time of diagnosis, high-risk populations need to be identified and cost-effective strategies for screening and early detection need to be developed. Early diagnostic biomarkers of gastric cancer could be useful for low-risk groups.

REFERENCES

1. Levine MS, Megibow AJ, and Kochman ML. Carcinoma of the stomach and duodenum. In Gore RM and Levine MS eds., *Textbook of Gastrointestinal Radiology*, 3rd edn. Philadelphia, PA: WB Saunders, 2008; pp. 619–44.

2. Lim JS *et al.* CT and PET in stomach cancer: preoperative staging and monitoring of response to therapy. *Radiographics* 2006; **26**: 143–56.

3. Mansfield PF. Clinical aspects and management of gastric carcinoma: management options: potentially respectable gastric cancer. In Abbruzzese JL, Evans DB, and Willett CG eds., *Gastrointestinal Oncology*. Oxford University Press, 2004; pp. 302–10.

4. Mulholland MW. Gastric neoplasms. In Mulholland MW and Lillimoe KD eds., *Greenfield's Surgery*. Philadelphia, PA: Lippincott Williams and Wilkins, 2006; pp. 743–55.

5. Sugano K. Gastric cancer: pathogenesis, screening, and treatment. *Gastrointest Endoscop Clin N Am* 2008; **18**: 513–22.

6. Houghton JM and Wang TC. Tumors of the stomach. In Feldman M, Friedman LS, and Sleisenger MH eds., *Gastrointestinal and Liver Diseases*, 8th edn. Philadelphia, PA: WB Saunders, 2006; pp. 1139–72.

7. Waxman I and Parmar KS. Clinical aspects and management of gastric carcinoma: diagnostic and staging procedures. In Abbruzzese JL, Evans DB, and Willett CG eds., *Gastrointestinal Oncology*. Oxford University Press, 2004; pp. 294–301.

8. Kurtz RC. Clinical aspects of gastric cancer. In Rustgi AK ed., *Gastrointestinal Cancers*. Edinburgh: WB Saunders, 2003; pp. 291–8.

9. Gore RM. Multidetector-row computed tomography of the gastrointestinal tract: principles of interpretation. In Gore RM and Levine MS eds., *Textbook of Gastrointestinal Radiology*, 3rd edn. Philadelphia, PA: WB Saunders, 2008; pp. 81–90.

10. Low RN. Magnetic resonance imaging of the hollow viscera. In Gore RM and Levine MS eds., *Textbook of Gastrointestinal Radiology*, 3rd edn. Philadelphia, PA: WB Saunders, 2008; pp. 91–106.

11. Low RN. Magnetic resonance imaging in the oncology patient: evaluation of the extrahepatic abdomen. *Semin Ultrasound CT MR* 2005; **26**: 224–36.

12. Low RN and Gurney J. Diffusion-weighted MRI (DWI) in the oncology patient: value of breath-hold DWI compared to unenhanced and gadolinium-enhanced MRI. *J Magn Reson Imaging* 2007; **25**: 848–58.

13. Gore RM. Endoscopic ultrasound. In Gore RM and Levine MS eds., *Textbook of Gastrointestinal Radiology*, 3rd edn. Philadelphia, PA: WB Saunders, 2008; pp. 177–82.

14. Aabakkaen L. Endoscopic diagnosis and treatment of gastric tumors. *Endsocopy* 2007; **39**: 974–7.

15. Jones DB. Role of endoscopic ultrasound in staging upper gastrointestinal cancers. *ANZ J Surg* 2007; **77**: 166–72.

16. Chen J, Cheong JH, Yun MJ *et al.* Improvement in preoperative staging of gastric adenocarcinoma with positron emission tomography. *Cancer* 2005; **103**(11): 2383–90.

17. Schmidt GP, Kramer H, Reiser MF *et al.* Whole-body magnetic resonance imaging and positron emission tomography-computed tomography in oncology. *Top Magn Reson Imaging* 2007; **18**: 193–202.

18. Weber WA and Ott K. Imaging of esophageal and gastric cancer. *Semin Oncol* 2004; **31**: 530–41.

19. Muruyama M. Early gastrointestinal cancers. *Abdom Imaging* 2003; **28**: 456–63.

20. Liakos T and Roukos DH. Challenges and promises towards personalized treatment of gastric cancer. *Ann Surg Oncol* 2008; **15**: 956–60.

21. Nitti D, Mocellin S, Marchet A *et al.* Recent advances in conventional and molecular prognostic factors for gastric carcinoma. *Surg Oncol Clin N Am* 2008; **17**: 467–83.

22. Fenoglio-Preiser C, Noffsinger A, and Stemmermann G. Pathology and natural history of gastric cancer. In Abbruzzese JL, Evans DB, and Willett CG eds., *Gastrointestinal Oncology*. Oxford University Press, 2004; pp. 281–93.

23. Lauers GY. Epithelial neoplasms of the stomach. In Odze RD, Goldblum JR, and Crawford JM eds., *Surgical Pathology of the GI Tract, Liver, Biliary Tract, and Pancreas*. Philadelphia, PA: WB Saunders, 2004; pp. 409–28.

24. Lauwers GY and Schimizu M. Pathology of gastric cancer. In Rustgi AK ed., *Gastrointestinal Cancers*. Edinburgh: WB Saunders, 2003; pp. 321–30.

25. McKinlay AW and El-Omar EM. Stomach: adenocarcinoma. In Weinstein WM, Hawkey CJ, and Bosch J eds., *Clinical Gastroenterology and Hepatology*. Philadelphia, PA: Elsevier-Mosby, 2005; pp. 233–42.

26. Monig SP *et al.* Staging of gastric cancer: correlation of lymph node size and metastatic infiltration. *AJR Am J Roentgenol* 1999; **173**: 365–7.

27. Kwee RM and Kwee TC. Imaging in local staging of gastric cancer: a systematic review. *J Clin Oncol* 2008; **25**: 2107–16.

28. Barry JD *et al.* Special interest radiology improves the perceived preoperative stage of gastric cancer. *Clin Radiol* 2002; **57**: 984–8.

29. Jensen EH and Tuttle TM. Preoperative staging and postoperative surveillance for gastric cancer. *Surg Clin North Am* 2007; **16**: 329–42.

30. Sasako M. Gastric cancer: surgical and adjuvant chemotherapy. *J Clin Oncol* 2008; **13**: 193–205.

31. Memon MA, Khan S, Yunus RM *et al.* Meta-analysis of laparoscopic and open distal gastrectomy for gastric carcinoma. *Surg Endosc* 2008; **22**: 1781–9.

32. Gore RM and Meyers MA. Pathways of abdominal disease spread. In Gore RM and Levine MS eds., *Textbook of Gastrointestinal Radiology*, 3rd edn. Philadelphia, PA: WB Saunders, 2008; pp. 2099–118.

33. Gore RM, Newmark GM, and Gore MD. Ascites and peritoneal fluid collections. In Gore RM and Levine MS eds., *Textbook of Gastrointestinal Radiology*, 3rd edn. Philadelphia, PA: WB Saunders, 2008; pp. 2119–34.

34. Gore RM and Miller FH. Stomach cancer. In Bragg DG, Rubin P, and Hricak H eds., *Oncologic Imaging*, 2nd edn. Philadelphia, PA: WB Saunders, 2002; pp. 391–418.

35. Wu B, Min P-Q, and Yang K. Utility of multidetector CT in the diagnosis of gastric bare area invasion by proximal gastric carcinoma. *Abdom Imaging* 2007; **32**: 264–89.

36. Farrell JJ and Wang TC. Biology of gastric cancer. In Rustgi AK ed., *Gastrointestinal Cancers*. Edinburgh: WB Saunders, 2003; pp. 299–320.

37. Ros PR and Erturk SM. Malignant tumors of the liver. In Gore RM and Levine MA eds., *Textbook of Gastrointestinal Radiology*, 3rd edn. Philadelphia, PA: WB Saunders, 2008; pp. 1623–62.

38. Low RN. MR imaging of the peritoneal spread of malignancy [review]. *Abdom Imaging* 2007; **32**(3): 267–83.

39. De Gaetano AM, Calcagni ML, Rufini V *et al.* Imaging of peritoneal carcinomatosis with FDG PET-CT: diagnostic patterns, case examples and pitfalls. *Abdom Imaging* 2008; Apr 30. (Epub ahead of print.)

40. Ba-Ssalamah A *et al.* Dedicated multidetector CT of the stomach: spectrum of disease. *Radiographics* 2003; **23**: 625–44.

41. Horton KM and Fishman EK. Current role of CT in imaging of the stomach. *Radiographics* 2003; **23**: 75–87.

42. Insko EK, Levine MS, Birnbaum BA, and Jacobs JE. Benign and malignant lesions of the stomach: evaluation of CT criteria for differentiation. *Radiology* 2003; **228**: 166–71.

43. Kim SH *et al.* Effect of adjusted positioning on gastric distension and fluid distribution during CT gastrography. *AJR Am J Roentgenol* 2005; **185**: 1180–4.

44. Kumano S, Murakami T, Kim T *et al.* T staging of gastric cancer: role of multi-detector row CT. *Radiology* 2005; **237**: 961–6.

45. Yang DM *et al.* 64 multidetector-row computed tomography for preoperative evaluation of gastric cancer: histological correlation. *J Comput Assist Tomogr* 2007; **31**: 98–103.

46. Chen B-B *et al.* Preoperative diagnosis of gastric tumors by three-dimensional multidetector row CT and double contrast barium meal study: correlation with surgical and histologic results. *J Formos Med Assoc* 2007; **106**: 943–52.

47. Matsuki M *et al.* Virtual CT gastrectomy by three-dimensional imaging using multidetector-row CT for laparoscopic gastrectomy. *Abdom Imaging* 2006; **31**: 268–76.

48. Matsuki M *et al.* Dual-phase 3D CT angiography during a single breath-hold using 16-MDCT: assessment of vascular anatomy before laparoscopic gastrectomy. *AJR Am J Roentgenol* 2006; **186**: 1079–85.

49. Callaway MP and Bailey D. Staging computed tomography in upper GI malignancy. A survey of the 5 cancer networks covered by the South West Cancer Intelligence Service. *Clin Radiol* 2005; **60**: 794–800.

50. Chen C-Y *et al.* Differentiation of gastric ulcers with MDCT. *Abdom Imaging* 2007; **32**: 688–93.

51. Pickhardt PJ and Asher DB. Wall thickening of the gastric antrum as a normal finding: multidetector CT with cadaveric comparison. *AJR Am J Roentgenol* 2003; **181**: 973–9.

52. Lee JH *et al.* Advanced gastric carcinoma with signet ring cell carcinoma versus non-signet ring cell carcinoma: differentiation with multidetector CT. *J Comput Assist Tomogr* 2006; **30**: 880–4.

53. Rossi M *et al.* Local invasion of gastric cancer: CT findings and pathologic correlation using 5-mm incremental scanning, hypotonia, and water filling. *AJR Am J Roentgenol* 1999; **172**: 383–8.

54. Shin KS *et al.* Three-dimensional MDCT gastrography compared with axial CT for the detection of early gastric cancer. *J Comput Assist Tomogr* 2007; **31**: 741–9.

55. Shimizu K *et al.* Diagnosis of gastric cancer with MDCT using the water-filling method and multiplanar reconstruction: CT-histologic correlation. *AJR Am J Roentgenol* 2005; **185**: 1152–8.

56. Kim YN *et al.* Gastric cancer staging at isotropic MDCT including coronal and sagittal MPR images: endoscopically diagnosed early vs. advanced gastric cancer. *Abdom Imaging* 2009; **34**: 26–34.

57. Hur J *et al.* Diagnostic accuracy of multidetector row computed tomography in T- and N staging of gastric cancer with histopathologic correlation. *J Comput Assist Tomogr* 2006; **30**: 372–7.

58. Kim HJ *et al.* Gastric cancer staging at multi-detector row CT gastrography: comparison of transverse and volumetric CT scanning. *Radiology* 2005; **236**: 879–85.

59. Chen C-Y, Wu D-C, Kang W-Y, and Hsu J-S. Staging of gastric cancer with 16-channel MDCT. *Abdom Imaging* 2006; **31**: 514–20.

60. Kumano S *et al.* Preoperative evaluation of perigastric vascular anatomy by 3-dimensional computed tomographic angiography using 16-channel multidetector-row computed tomography for laparoscopic gastrectomy in patients with early gastric cancer. *J Comput Assist Tomogr* 2007; **31**: 93–7.

61. Monig SP, Zirbes TK, Schroder W *et al.* Staging of gastric cancer: correlation of lymph node size and metastatic infiltration. *AJR Am J Roentgenol* 1999; **173**: 365–7.

62. Choi HJ *et al.* Contrast-enhanced CT for differentiation of ovarian metastasis from gastrointestinal tract cancer: stomach cancer versus colon cancer. *AJR Am J Roentgenol* 2006; **187**: 1873–7.

63. Chen C-Y *et al.* Gastric cancer: preoperative local staging with 3D multi-detector row CT. Correlation with surgical and histopathology results. *Radiology* 2007; **242**: 472–82.

64. Kim JH *et al.* Diagnostic performance of virtual gastroscopy using MDCT in early gastric cancer compared with 2D axial CT: focusing on interobserver variation. *AJR Am J Roentgenol* 2007; **188**: 299–305.

65. Kim JH *et al.* Imaging of various gastric lesions with 2D MPR and CT gastrography performed with multidetector CT. *Radiographics* 2006; **26**: 1101–8.

66. Chen C-Y *et al.* MDCT for differentiation of category T1 and T2 malignant lesions from benign gastric ulcers. *AJR Am J Roentgenol* 2008; **190**: 1505–11.

67. Kim AY, Kim HJ, and Ha HK. Gastric cancer by multidetector row CT: preoperative staging. *Abdom Imaging* 2005; **30**: 465–72.

68. Wei W-Z *et al.* Evaluation of contrast-enhanced helical hydro-CT in staging gastric cancer. *World J Gastroenterol* 2005; **11**: 4592–5.

69. Kim JH, Park SH, Hong HS, and Auh YH. CT gastrography. *Abdom Imaging* 2005; **30**: 509–17.

70. Kim J-Y *et al.* Differentiating malignant from benign wall thickening in postoperative stomach using helical computed tomography: results of multivariate analysis. *J Comput Assist Tomogr* 2007; **31**: 455–62.

71. Kim JH *et al.* Early gastric cancer: virtual gastroscopy. *Abdom Imaging* 2006; **31**: 507–13.

72. Kim YN, Choi D, Kim SH *et al.* Gastric cancer staging at isotropic MDCT including coronal and sagittal MRP images: endoscopically diagnosed early vs. advanced gastric cancer. *Abdom Imaging* 2009; **34**: 26–34.

73. Matsui H *et al.* Relatively small size linitis plastica of the stomach: multislice CT detection of tissue fibrosis. *Abdom Imaging* 2007; **32**: 694–7.

74. Yu J-S *et al.* Value of nonvisualized primary lesions of gastric cancer on preoperative MDCT. *AJR Am J Roentgenol* 2007; **189**: W315–19.

75. Bentrem D *et al.* Clinical correlation of endoscopic ultrasonography with pathologic stage and outcome in patients undergoing curative resection for gastric cancer. *Ann Surg Oncol* 2007; **14**: 1853–9.

76. Prasad P, Wittmann J, and Pereira SP. Endoscopic ultrasound of the upper gastrointestinal tract and mediastinum: diagnosis and therapy. *Cardiovasc Intervent Radiol* 2006; **29**: 947–57.

77. Habermann CR *et al.* Preoperative staging of gastric adenocarcinoma: comparison of helical CT and endoscopic ultrasound. *Radiology* 2004; **230**: 465–71.

78. Yoshida S *et al.* Diagnostic ability of high-frequency ultrasound probe sonography in staging early gastric cancer, especially for submucosal invasion. *Abdom Imaging* 2005; **30**: 518–32.

79. Talamonti M. Endoscopic ultrasound for gastric cancer: a technique for preoperative risk stratification in need of further refinements. *Ann Surg Oncol* 2007; **14**: 3293–4.

80. Kwee RM and Kwee TC. The accuracy of endoscopic ultrasonography in differentiating mucosal from deeper gastric cancer. *Am J Gastroenterol* 2008; **103**: 1801–9.

81. Park SR *et al.* Endoscopic ultrasound and computed tomography in restaging and predicting prognosis after neoadjuvant chemotherapy in patients with locally advanced gastric cancer. *Cancer* 2008; **112**: 2368–76.

82. Arocena MG *et al.* MRI and endoscopic ultrasonography in the staging of gastric cancer. *Rev Esp Enferm Dig* 2006; **98**: 582–90.

83. Gore RM. Endoscopic ultrasound. In Gore RM and Levine MD eds., *Textbook of Gastrointestinal Radiology*, 3rd edn. Philadelphia, PA: WB Saunders, 2008; pp. 167–72.

84. Puli SR, Reddi J, Bechtold ML *et al.* How good is endoscopic ultrasound for TNM staging of gastric cancers? A meta-analysis and systematic review. *World J Gastroenterol* 2006; **14**: 4011–19.

85. Blodgett TM, McCook BM, and Federle MP. Positron emission computed tomography/computed tomography: protocol issues and options. *Semin Nuclear Med* 2006; **36**: 157–68.

86. Ono K *et al.* The detection rates and tumor clinical/pathological stages of whole-body FDG-PET cancer screening. *Ann Nucl Med* 2007; **21**: 65–72.

87. Dehdashti F and Siegel B. Neoplasms of the esophagus and stomach. *Semin Nucl Med* 2004; **34**: 198–208.

88. Rosenbaum SJ *et al.* Staging and follow-up of gastrointestinal tumors with PET/CT. *Abdom Imaging* 2006; **31**: 25–35.

89. Zhu Z *et al.* Improving evaluation of primary gastric malignancies by distending the stomach with milk immediately before 18F-FDG PET scanning. *J Nucl Med Technol* 2008; **36**: 25–9.

90. van Vliet EPM *et al.* Radiologist experience and CT examination quality determine metastasis detection in patients with esophageal or gastric cardia cancer. *Eur Radiol* 2008; **18**: 2475–84.

91. Herrmann K *et al.* Imaging gastric cancer with PET and radiotracers 18F-FLT and 18F-FDG: a comparative analysis. *J Nucl Med* 2007; **48**: 1945–50.

92. Jin H and Min P-Q. Computed tomography of gastrocolic ligament: involvement in malignant tumors of the stomach. *Abdom Imaging* 2007; **32**: 59–65.

93. Chen J *et al.* Improvement in preoperative staging of gastric adenocarcinoma with positron emission tomography. *Cancer* 2005; **103**: 2383–90.

94. Yun M, Lim JS, Noh SH *et al.* Lymph node staging of gastric cancer using (18)F-FDG PET: a comparison with CT. *J Nucl Med* 2005; **46**: 1582–8.

95. Kim S-K *et al.* Assessment of lymph node metastases using 18F-FDG PET in patients with advanced gastric cancer. *Eur J Nucl Med Mol Imaging* 2006; **33**: 148–55.

96. Mukai K *et al.* Usefulness of preoperative FDG-PET for detection of gastric cancer. *Gastric Cancer* 2006; **9**: 192–6.

97. Yang Q-M, Bando E, Kawamura T *et al.* The diagnostic value of PET-CT for peritoneal dissemination of abdominal malignancies. *Jpn J Cancer Chemother* 2006; **33**: 1817–21.

98. Lim JS *et al.* Comparison of CT and 18F-FDG PET for detecting peritoneal metastasis on the preoperative evaluation for gastric carcinoma. *Korean J Radiol* 2006; **7**: 249–56.

99. Park MJ *et al.* Detecting recurrence of gastric cancer: the value of FDG PET/CT. *Abdom Imaging* 2009; **34**: 441–7.

100. Lim JS *et al.* CT and PET in stomach cancer: preoperative staging and monitoring of response to therapy. *Radiographics* 2006; **26**: 143–56.

101. Ben-Haim S and Ell P. 18F-FDG PET and PET/CT in the evaluation of cancer treatment response. *J Nucl Med* 2009; **50**: 88–99.

102. Nakamoto Y, Togashi K, Kaneta T *et al.* Clinical value of whole-body FDG-PET for recurrent gastric cancer: a multicenter study. *Jpn J Clin Oncol* 2009; **39**: 297–302.

103. Kim AY *et al.* MRI in staging advanced gastric cancer: is it useful compared with spiral CT? *J Comput Assist Tomogr* 2000; **24**: 389–94.

104. Motohara T and Semelka RC. MRI in staging of gastric cancer. *Abdom Imaging* 2002; **27**: 376–83.

105. Heye T *et al*. New coil concept for endoluminal MR imaging: initial results in staging of gastric carcinoma in correlation with histopathology. *Eur Radiol* 2006; **16**: 2401–9.

106. Palmowski M *et al*. Magnetic resonance imaging for local staging of gastric carcinoma: results of an in vitro study. *J Comput Assist Tomogr* 2006; **30**: 896–902.

107. Lubienski A *et al*. MR imaging of gastric wall layers in vitro: correlation to the histologic wall structure. *Rofo* 2002; **174**: 490–4.

108. Sohn KM *et al*. Comparing MR imaging and CT in staging of gastric carcinoma. *AJR Am J Roentgenol* 2000; **174**: 1551–7.

109. Matsushiata M *et al*. Extraserosal invasion in advanced gastric cancer: evaluation with MR imaging. *Radiology* 1994; **22**: 35–40.

110. Sato C *et al*. MR imaging of gastric cancer in vitro: accuracy of invasion depth diagnosis. *Eur Radiol* 2004; **14**: 1543–9.

111. Tatsumi Y *et al*. Preoperative diagnosis of lymph node metastases in gastric cancer by magnetic resonance imaging with ferumoxtran-10. *Gastric Cancer* 2006; **9**: 120–8.

112. Lee SM *et al*. Usefulness of CT volumetry for primary gastric lesions in predicting pathologic response to neoadjuvant chemotherapy in advanced gastric cancer. *Abdom Imaging* 2009; **34**: 430–40.

113. Nakajima T. Gastric cancer treatment guidelines in Japan. *Gastric Cancer* 2002; **5**: 1–5.

114. Minsky BD. Chemotherapy and radiation therapy of gastric cancer. In Rustgi AK ed., *Gastrointestinal Cancers*. Edinburgh: WB Saunders, 2003; pp. 345–54.

115. Gunderson L and Sosin H. Adenocarcinoma of the stomach: areas of failure in reoperation series: clinicopathologic correlation and implications for adjuvant therapy. *Int J Radiat Biol Phys* 1982; **8**: 1–11.

116. Roviello F, Marrelli D, de Manzoni G *et al*. Prospective study of peritoneal recurrence after curative surgery for gastric cancer. *Br J Surg* 2003; **90**: 1113–19.

117. Maehara Y, Hasuda S, Koga T *et al*. Postoperative outcome and sites of recurrence in patients following curative resection of gastric cancer. *Br J Surg* 2000; **87**: 353–7.

118. Whiting J, Sano T, Saka M *et al*. Follow-up of gastric cancer: a review. *Gastric Cancer* 2006; **9**: 74–81.

119. Yoo CH, Noh SH, Shin DW *et al*. Recurrence following curative resection for gastric carcinoma. *Br J Surg* 2000; **87**: 236–42.

120. Kodera Y, Ito S, Yamamura Y *et al*. Follow-up surveillance for recurrence of early gastric cancer lacks survival benefit. *Ann Surg Oncol* 2003; **10**: 898–902.

121. MacDonald JA, Smalley SR, Benedetti J *et al*. Chemoradiotherapy after surgery compared with surgery alone for adenocarcinoma of the stomach or gastroesophageal junction. *New Engl J Med* 2001; **345**: 725–30.

122. Hironaka SI, Boku N, Ohtsu A *et al*. Sequential methotrexate and 5-fluorouracil therapy for gastric cancer patients with bone metastasis. *Gastric Cancer* 2003; **3**: 19–23.

123. Moehler M, Lyros O, Gockel I *et al.* Multidisciplinary management of gastric and gastroesopha-geal cancer. *World J Gastroenterol* 2008; **14**: 3773–80.

124. Wotherspoon A and Dogan A. Gastric lymphoma. In Weinstein WM, Hawkey CJ and Bosch J eds., *Clinical Gastroenterology and Hepatology*. Philadelphia, PA: Elsevier-Mosby, 2005; pp. 243–6.

125. Wallace MB and Thomas CR. Gastrointestinal lymphomas and AIDS related gastrointes-tinal cancers. In Rustgi AK ed., *Gastrointestinal Cancers*. Edinburgh: WB Saunders, 2003; pp. 655–80.

126. Luk GD. Tumors of the stomach. In Feldman M, Scharschmidt BF, and Sleisenger MH eds., *Gastrointestinal and Liver Disease*, 6th edn. Philadelphia, PA: WB Saunders, 1998; pp. 733–60.

127. Sepulveda AR. Mucosa-associated lymphoid tissue lymphomas. In Abbruzzese JL, Evans DB, Willett CG, and Fenoglio-Preiser C eds., *Gastrointestinal Oncology*. New York: Oxford University Press, 2004; pp. 803–11.

128. Cabanillas F and Pro B. Low- and high- grade lymphomas. In Abbruzzese JL, Evans DB, Willett CG and Fenoglio-Preiser C eds., *Gastrointestinal Oncology*. New York: Oxford University Press, 2004; pp. 812–20.

129. Park SH, Han JK, Kim TK *et al.* Unusual gastric tumors: radiologic-pathologic correlation. *Radiographics* 1999; **196**: 1435–46.

130. Kim YH, Lim HK, Han JK *et al.* Low-grade gastric mucosa-associated lymphoid tissue lymph-oma: correlation of radiographic and pathologic findings. *Radiology* 1999; **212**: 241–8.

131. Park MS, Kim KW, Yu JS *et al.* Radiographic findings of primary B-cell lymphoma of the stom-ach: low-grade versus high-grade malignancy in relation to the mucosa-associated lymphoid tissue concept. *AJR Am J Roentgenol* 2002; **179**: 1297–304.

132. Kessar P, Norton A, Rohatiner AZ *et al.* CT appearances of mucosa-associated lymphoid tissue (MALT) lymphoma. *Eur Radiol* 1999; **9**: 693–6.

133. Brown JA, Carson BW, Gascoyne RD *et al.* Low grade gastric MALT lymphoma: radiographic findings. *Clin Radiol* 2000; **55**: 384–9.

134. An SK, Han JK, Kim YH *et al.* Gastric mucosa-associated lymphoid tissue lymphoma: spec-trum of findings at double-contrast gastrointestinal examination with pathologic correlation. *Radiographics* 2001; **21**: 1491–502.

135. Choi D, Lim HK, Lee SJ *et al.* Gastric mucosa-associated lymphoid tissue lymphoma: helical CT findings and pathologic correlation. *AJR Am J Roentgenol* 2002; **178**: 1117–22.

136. Byun JH, Ha HK, Kim AY *et al.* CT findings in peripheral T-cell lymphoma involving the gastrointestinal tract. *Radiology* 2003; **227**: 59–67.

137. Lee DH. Two-dimensional and three-dimensional imaging of gastric tumors using spiral CT. *Abdom Imaging* 2000; **25**(1): 1–6.

138. Gossios K, Katsimbri P, and Tsianos E. CT features of gastric lymphoma. *Eur Radiol* 2000; **10**: 425–30.

139. Scarpa M, Bertin M, Ruffolo C *et al.* A systematic review on the clinical diagnosis of gastrointestinal stromal tumors. *J Surg Oncol* 2008; **98**: 384–92.

140. Davila RE and Faigel DO. Gastrointestinal stromal tumors and gastroduodenal carcinoid tumors. In Weinstein WM, Hawkey CJ, and Bosch J eds., *Clinical Gastroenterology and Hepatology*. Philadelphia, PA: Elsevier-Mosby, 2005; pp. 247–52.

141. Keohan ML, Hibshoosh H, and Antman KH. Gastrointestinal sarcomas. In Rustgi AK ed., *Gastrointestinal Cancers*. Edinburgh: WB Saunders, 2003; pp. 681–720.

142. Hueman MT and Schulick RD. Management of gastrointestinal stromal tumors. *Surg Clin North Am* 2008; **88**: 599–614.

143. Iwahashi M, Takifuji K, Ojima T *et al.* Surgical management of small gastrointestinal stromal tumors of the stomach. *World J Surg* 2006; **30**: 28–35.

144. Joensuu H. Risk stratification of patients diagnosed with gastrointestinal stromal tumor. *Hum Pathol* 2008; **39**: 1411–19.

145. Bertolini V, Chiaravalli AM, Klersy C *et al.* Gastrointestinal stromal tumors – frequency, malignancy, and new prognostic factors: the experience of a single institution. *Pathol Res Pract* 2008; **204**: 219–33.

146. Vallböhmer D, Marcus HE, Baldus SE *et al.* Serosal penetration is an important prognostic factor for gastrointestinal stromal tumors. *Oncol Rep* 2008; **20**: 779–83.

147. Canda AE, Ozsoy Y, Nalbant OA, and Sagol O. Gastrointestinal stromal tumor of the stomach with lymph node metastasis. *World J Surg Oncol* 2008; **5**: 97–102.

148. Catena F, Di Battista M, Fusaroli P *et al.* Laparoscopic treatment of gastric GIST: report of 21 cases and literature's review. *J Gastrointest Surg* 2008; **12**: 561–8.

149. Burkill GJ, Badran M, Al-Muderis O *et al.* Malignant gastrointestinal stromal tumor: distribution, imaging features, and pattern of metastatic spread. *Radiology* 2003; **226**: 527–32.

150. Darnell A, Dalmau E, Pericay C *et al.* Gastrointestinal stromal tumors. *Abdom Imaging* 2006; **31**: 387–99.

151. Horton KM, Juluru K, Montogomery E, and Fishman EK. Computed tomography imaging of gastrointestinal stromal tumors with pathology correlation. *J Comput Assist Tomogr* 2004; **28**: 811–17.

152. Kim HC, Lee JM, Choi SH *et al.* Imaging of gastrointestinal stromal tumors. *J Comput Assist Tomogr* 2004; **28**: 596–604.

153. Kim HC, Lee JM, Kim KW *et al.* Gastrointestinal stromal tumors of the stomach: CT findings a prediction of malignancy. *AJR Am J Roentgenol* 2004; **183**: 893–8.

154. Lee MW, Kim SH, Kim YJ *et al.* Gastrointestinal stromal tumor of the stomach: preliminary results of preoperative evaluation with CT gastrography. *Abdom Imaging* 2008; **33**: 255–61.

155. Kim HC, Lee JM, Kim SH *et al.* Small gastrointestinal stromal tumours with focal areas of low attenuation on CT: pathological correlation. *Clin Radiol* 2005; **60**: 384–8.

156. Chatzipantelis P, Salla C, Karoumpalis I *et al.* Endoscopic ultrasound-guided fine needle aspiration biopsy in the diagnosis of gastrointestinal stromal tumors of the stomach: a study of 17 cases. *J Gastrointest Liver Dis* 2008; **17**: 15–20.

157. Ghanem N, Altehoefer C, Furtwängler A *et al.* Computed tomography in gastrointestinal stromal tumors. *Eur Radiol* 2003; **13**: 1669–78.

158. O'Sullivan PJ, Harris AC, Ho SG, and Munk PL. The imaging features of gastrointestinal stromal tumours. *Eur J Radiol* 2006; **60**: 431–8.

159. Sharp RM, Ansel HJ, and Keel SB. Best cases from the AFIP: gastrointestinal stromal tumor. *Radiographics* 2001; **21**: 1557–60.

160. Gong JS, Zuo M, Yang P *et al.* Value of CT in the diagnosis and follow-up of gastrointestinal stromal tumors. *Clin Imaging* 2008; **32**: 172–7.

161. Tateishi U, Miyake M, Maeda T *et al.* CT and MRI findings in KIT-weak or KIT-negative atypical gastrointestinal stromal tumors. *Eur Radiol* 2006; **16**: 1537–43.

162. Sandrasegaran K, Rajesh A, Rushing DA *et al.* Gastrointestinal stromal tumors: CT and MRI findings. *Eur Radiol* 2005; **15**: 1407–14.

163. Ulusan S, Koc Z and Kayaselcuk F. Gastrointestinal stromal tumours: CT findings. *Br J Radiol* 2008; **81**: 618–23.

164. Cegarra-Navarro MF, de la Calle MA, Girela-Baena E *et al.* Ruptured gastrointestinal stromal tumors: radiologic findings in six cases. *Abdom Imaging* 2005; **30**: 535–42.

165. Tateishi U, Hasegawa T, Satake M, and Moriyama N. Gastrointestinal stromal tumor. Correlation of computed tomography findings with tumor grade and mortality. *J Comput Assist Tomogr* 2003; **27**: 792–8.

166. Bechtold RE, Chen MY, Stanton CA *et al.* Cystic changes in hepatic and peritoneal metastases from gastrointestinal stromal tumors treated with Gleevec. *Abdom Imaging* 2003; **28**: 808–14.

167. Holdsworth CH, Badawi RD, Manola JB *et al.* CT and PET: early prognostic indicators of response to imatinib mesylate in patients with gastrointestinal stromal tumor. *AJR Am J Roentgenol* 2007; **189**: 324–30.

168. Lassau N, Lamuraglia M, Chami L *et al.* Gastrointestinal stromal tumors treated with imatinib: monitoring response with contrast-enhanced sonography. *AJR Am J Roentgenol* 2006; **187**: 1267–73.

169. Vanel D, Albiter M, Shapeero L *et al.* Role of computed tomography in the follow-up of hepatic and peritoneal metastases of GIST under imatinib mesylate treatment: a prospective study of 54 patients. *Eur J Radiol* 2005; **54**: 118–23.

170. Hong X, Choi H, Loyer EM *et al.* Gastrointestinal stromal tumor: role of CT in diagnosis and in response evaluation and surveillance after treatment with imatinib. *Radiographics* 2006; **26**: 481–95.

171. Van den Abbeele AD. The lessons of GIST – PET and PET/CT: a new paradigm for imaging. *Oncologist* 2008; **13** (Suppl 2): 8–13.

172. Kitamura Y. Gastrointestinal stromal tumors: past, present, and future. *J Gastroenterol* 2008; **43**: 499–508.

173. Nakamori M, Iwahashi M, Nakamura M *et al.* Laparoscopic resection for gastrointestinal stromal tumors of the stomach. *Am J Surg* 2008; **196**: 425–9.

174. Shankar S, van Sonnenberg E, Desai J *et al.* Gastrointestinal stromal tumor. New nodule-within-in-a-mass pattern of recurrence after partial response to imatinib mesylate. *Radiology* 2005; **235**: 892–8.

175. Warakaulle DR and Gleeson F. MDCT appearance of gastrointestinal stromal tumors after therapy with imatinib mesylate. *AJR Am J Roentgenol* 2006; **186**: 510–15.

176. Yang DM, Kim H, Kang JH *et al.* Computed tomography and sonographic findings of hepatic metastases from gastrointestinal stromal tumors after chemotherapy. *J Comput Assist Tomogr* 2005; **29**: 592–5.

177. Mabille M, Vanel D, Albiter M *et al.* Follow-up of hepatic and peritoneal metastases of GIST under imatinib therapy requires different criteria of radiologic evaluation (size is not everything!!!). *Eur J Radiol* 2009; **69**(2): 204–8.

178. Yao JC and Ajani JA. Management of neuroendocrine cancers of the gastrointestinal tract: carcinoid tumors. In Abbruzzese JL, Evans DB, Willett CG, and Fenoglio-Preiser C eds., *Gastrointestinal Oncology*. New York: Oxford University Press, 2004; pp. 773–9.

179. Metz DC and Jensen RT. Endocrine tumors of the gastrointestinal tract. In Rustgi AK ed., *Gastrointestinal Cancers*. Edinburgh: WB Saunders, 2003; pp. 681–720.

180. Rindi G, Luinetti O, Cornaggia M, Capaella C, and Solcia E. Three subtypes of gastric argyrophil carcinoid and the gastric neuroendocrine carcinoma: a clinicopathologic study. *Gastroenterology* 1993; **104**: 994–1006.

181. Rindi G, Bordi C, Rappel S, La Rosa S, Stolte M, and Solcia E. Gastric carcinoids and neuroendocrine carcinomas: pathogenesis, pathology, and behavior. *World J Surg* 1996; **20**: 168–72.

182. Binstock AJ, Johnson CD, Stephens DH *et al.* Carcinoid tumors of the stomach: a clinical and radiographic study. *AJR Am J Roentgenol* 2001; **176**: 947–51.

183. Levy AD and Sobin LH. Gastrointestinal carcinoids: imaging features with clinicopathologic comparison. *Radiographics* 2007; **27**: 237–57.

184. Buck JL and Sobin LH. Carcinoids of the gastrointestinal tract. *Radiographics* 1990; **10**: 1081–95.

185. Berger MW and Stephens DH. Gastric carcinoid tumors associated with chronic hypergastrinemia in a patient with Zollinger-Ellison syndrome. *Radiology* 1996; **201**: 371–3.

186. Pelage JP, Soyer P, Boudiaf M *et al.* Carcinoid tumors of the abdomen: CT features. *Abdom Imaging* 1999; **24**: 240–5.

187. Chang S, Choi D, Lee SJ *et al.* Neuroendocrine neoplasms of the gastrointestinal tract: classification, pathologic basis and imaging features. *Radiographics* 2007; **27**: 1667–79.

188. Gupta R, Dastane A, McKenna RJ Jr., and Marchevsky AM. What can we learn from the errors in the frozen section diagnosis of gastric carcinoid tumors? An evidence-based approach. *Hum Pathol* 2009; **40**(1): 1–9.

8

Gastric cancer: current trends and future opportunities

Richard M. Gore, Huan Zhang, Chiao-Yun Chen, and Kenjiro Yasuda

Introduction

Napoleon Bonaparte's remarkable political and military career was ended by Wellington at Waterloo in 1815. He died at age 52 on St. Helena in 1821 due to gastric cancer. Napoleon had a childhood of poverty, a poor diet in his early career, and a strong family history of gastric cancer, all of which contributed to his demise. It is now apparent that *Helicobacter pylori*, acting in the context of host genetic susceptibility, is responsible for most cases of stomach cancer. Napoleon was most likely infected with *H. pylori* – an example of the bacterium being mightier than the sword. This interaction between bacterium and host offers a new paradigm for carcinogenesis in the gastrointestinal (GI) tract and provides clues to the prevention and screening of this lethal malignancy [1].

As information concerning the epidemiology and molecular genetics of gastric cancer improves, sophisticated strategies for early detection and prevention of this disease in high-risk areas of the world will be developed. Eventually, molecular techniques will help identify those people at highest risk for this disease, so that resource-intensive endoscopic screening programs can be directed to this population. It is possible that, with directed use, screening programs will be validated by gastric cancer mortality reduction [2].

In this chapter, new concepts and horizons concerning prevention, screening, diagnosis, and treatment of patients with gastric adenocarcinoma are presented.

Primary prevention

Diet

The main focus of primary prevention of gastric cancer is diet. It is advisable to reduce the intake of foods altered by smoking, pickling, salting, and other chemical preservatives. Agricultural methods can be modified to reduce the nitrate content of vegetables. The dramatic decrease in the incidence of gastric cancer in the United States is linked to dietary changes associated with improved transport of fresh produce, wide availability of fresh or frozen meat, and home refrigeration and freezing. The power of primary prevention is highlighted by changes in the quality of the food supply engendered by enhanced technology.

There is a strong association between high salt intake and risk of gastric cancer [3, 4]. The daily intake of sodium chloride, however, has decreased drastically in most Western countries and in Japan, in part due to public health campaigns to reduce hypertensive diseases. This may be at least partially responsible for declines in gastric cancer rates as well.

Epidemiologic evidence suggests that increased intake of fresh fruits and vegetables is associated with decreased gastric cancer rates [4]. This has been validated by numerous case–control and cohort studies of gastric cancer. Dietary indices of micronutrient intake have been calculated and indicate possible protective effects of beta-carotene and vitamin C or foods that contain these compounds. A chemoprevention trial in China reported a statistically significant reduction in gastric cancer mortality rate after supplementation with beta-carotene, vitamin E, and selenium [5]. The population studied, however, may have been nutritionally deficient, raising questions concerning the applicability of these results to other populations. Additionally, the experimental design did not permit assessment of the relative effects of beta-carotene, vitamin E, and selenium. In a randomized double-blind chemoprevention trial in Venezuela in a population at increased risk for gastric cancer, a combination of antioxidant vitamins (vitamins C, E, and beta-carotene) failed to modify the progression or regression of precancerous gastric lesions [6]. Another potential explanation for the lack of benefit of vitamin supplementation in this trial was the high prevalence of advanced premalignant lesions and of *Helicobacter pylori* infection [7].

A secondary analysis of the Alpha-Tocopherol Beta-Carotene trial conducted in male smokers in Finland evaluated the effect of supplementation on gastric cancer incidence [8]. No protective effects of these supplements against gastric cancer were observed. Six-year follow-up results of a study of 976 Colombian patients have been reported. Patients were randomly assigned to receive eight different treatments that included vitamin supplements and anti-*Helicobacter* therapy either alone or in combination versus placebo. In 79 patients who received anti-*Helicobacter* therapy, borderline regression of intestinal metaplasia when compared with a placebo (15% vs 6%; relative risk = 3.1; 95% confidence interval = 1.0–9.3) was noted. However, the combination of antibiotics and vitamins did not confer additional benefits. More importantly, the progression rates of intestinal metaplasia were comparable irrespective of the treatments received. The progression rate was 23% in the placebo group and 17% in antibiotic recipients [9].

Aspirin

Researchers have long speculated that non-steroidal anti-inflammatory drugs (NSAIDs) might reduce the risk for gastric and other types of cancer. In order to investigate this theory, researchers in Sweden conducted a population-based case–control study in five Swedish counties. The researchers interviewed 567 individuals with gastric cancer and 1165 control subjects. The participants were questioned regarding the use of pain relievers. The researchers found that aspirin users had a moderately reduced risk of gastric cancer when compared with the control group that never used NSAIDs. The risk of gastric cancer was reduced as the frequency of aspirin use increased. While the results indicated a relationship between aspirin and gastric cancer risk, they did not establish a clear association between gastric cancer risk and non-aspirin NSAIDs or other pain relievers. These investigators concluded that aspirin may play a role in reducing the risk of gastric cancer [9].

Helicobacter pylori eradication

Prevention of gastric cancer via eradication of *H. pylori* infection is being actively considered in several countries [10, 11, 12, 13, 14, 15]. Many questions remain unanswered concerning the natural history of *H. pylori* infection, including the mechanism of transmission and the rates of reinfection or recrudescence for different populations [16, 17]. Since nearly half of the world population is infected, antibacterial treatment seems impractical.

Vaccination against *H. pylori* is very effective in experimental animals, but thus far such efficacy has not been studied in humans. Prevention randomized trials are also under way and might soon indicate whether curing *H. pylori* infection reduces cancer rates or stops the progression of precancerous lesions.

A randomized clinical trial evaluating the effect of eradicating *H. pylori* infection was conducted in a high-risk area of China [10]. Otherwise healthy carriers of *H. pylori* were randomly assigned to either a 2-week course of antibiotic therapy with omeprazole, a combination of amoxicillin and clavulanate potassium, and metronidazole ($N = 817$), or placebo ($N = 813$). After a 7.5-year follow-up, gastric cancer was not reduced in the treatment arm (7 vs 11 cases; $P = 0.33$). In a subgroup analysis among those free of precancerous lesions at study entry, a statistically significant reduction in the development of gastric cancer was observed in the treatment arm compared with placebo (0 vs 6 cases; $P = 0.02$).

Although *H. pylori* can be successfully eradicated by antibiotics and proton pump inhibitors in most patients, increasing antibiotic resistance in the bacterium remains a serious problem. Accordingly, there is a strong rationale for the development of effective vaccines against *H. pylori* and over the last several years several approaches have been used to develop effective vaccines. Various routes of administration have been studied including oral, rectal, and intramuscular for mucosal immunization in mice. It appears that long-lasting protective immunity against *H. pylori* requires systemic and mucosal activation of T1 helper cells [18, 19, 20].

Screening

The value of screening asymptomatic individuals for gastric cancer remains controversial and unsettled. An effective screening program should have the following characteristics: the disease should be common in the population, otherwise the individual benefit will not offset the risk, cost, and inconvenience of screening the rest of the population; the diagnostic test(s) used should be safe, simple, inexpensive, and reliable; and effective treatment should be available [21, 22, 23, 24, 25, 26, 27, 28].

Mass screening programs have been implemented in some countries (e.g., Japan, Venezuela, and Chile) where there continues to be a high incidence of gastric cancer. By contrast, the relatively low incidence of gastric cancer in other regions (including the United States) makes this strategy less attractive. Proponents of gastric cancer screening in low-risk regions agree that case finding rather than mass screening is the most appropriate approach for early detection. Case finding is the testing of patients who have sought health care for disorders that may be unrelated to the chief complaint [21, 22, 23, 24, 25, 26, 27, 28].

Mass screening programs for gastric cancer using upper gastrointestinal barium studies have been available in Japan since 1960. The number of patients examined in 1985 was over five million and the number of gastric cancers detected was more than 6000. While half of these cancers were early gastric cancers, the gold standard of mortality reduction has not been demonstrated [1].

Gastroscopic examination has been proposed as a screening method for the early detection of gastric cancer. No randomized trials evaluating the impact of screening on mortality from gastric cancer have been reported, although a Japanese study randomizing municipalities within a prefecture is ongoing [21]. Time–trend analysis and case–control studies of gastric endoscopy suggest a twofold decrease in gastric cancer mortality in screened versus unscreened individuals [22, 23, 24, 25, 26]; however, this stands in contrast to studies of stronger design.

A cohort study of 24 134 individuals with a follow-up period of 40 months did not demonstrate a statistically significant decrease in gastric cancer mortality among men or women who were screened compared with those who were not screened [27]. A larger prospective study examined the association between screening in the previous 12 months and subsequent gastric cancer mortality and other-cause mortality. The risk of death from gastric cancer and from causes of death other than gastric cancer were reduced among those who had participated in gastric cancer screening programs, demonstrating a selection for healthier individuals into screening programs [28].

Another cohort study was conducted in Linqu County, China, where gastric cancer rates are high, in which over 4000 adult residents were screened. Individuals were screened at an average of 4.5-year intervals, except for a high-risk subset (689 individuals) who were screened 2 years after the initial examination. Of the 85 cases of gastric cancer occurring in the cohort, 58 were detected with screening. No impact on gastric cancer mortality was observed among screened individuals. The standardized mortality ratio (SMR) for gastric cancer 10 years after the initial screen was 1.01 (95% confidence interval, 0.72–1.37). The SMR for all-cause mortality was significantly lower among participants since individuals with hypertension, liver disease, and chronic obstructive pulmonary disease were not eligible to participate [29]. A screening study was begun in Venezuela in 1980, using radiographic fluorography [30]. The efficacy of this program in reducing mortality from stomach cancer was evaluated by means of a case–control study. Analyses determined that the tests were ineffective at reducing mortality from gastric cancer.

In Japan, measurement of serum pepsinogen (types I and II) levels in 5113 subjects also screened by endoscopy (13 gastric cancers detected) used cut-off points for identifying the risk for gastric cancer of less than 70 ng/ml for pepsinogen I and less than 3 for the type I:type II ratio. This combination provided a sensitivity of 84.6%, a specificity of 73.5%, a positive predictive value of 0.81%, and a negative predictive value of 99.6% [31].

There may be some justification for screening some populations of Americans at higher risk, although there is considerable discussion about how high the incidence rate would have to be in order to make the examination worthwhile. Potential subgroups might include elderly with atrophic gastritis or pernicious anemia, patients with partial gastrectomy [32], patients with the diagnosis of sporadic adenomas [33], familial adenomatous polyposis [34], hereditary nonpolyposis colon cancer [35], and immigrant ethnic populations from countries with high rates of gastric carcinoma [36, 37].

The requirements of cancer screening programs differ between countries due to differences in cancer incidence and mortality. Gastric cancer screening would not appear to be an optimal use of resources in North America, where the incidence of this disease is relatively low. Case finding in select high-risk groups may be more feasible [38].

Genetics

The suppression/inactivation of several tumor suppressor genes and the activation of several growth-promoting genes appear to be important in the pathogenesis of gastric cancer (Figure 8.1). At the present time, there is no clear "gate-keeper gene" similar to APC in colon cancer, and the precise time of the gene alterations in relation to the progression of gastric cancer remains to be defined. Several host genetic factors have recently been described and include polymorphisms in the genes for the proinflammatory cytokine interleukin-1β (IL-1β) and tumor necrosis factor-α (TNF-α). It appears that the effect of these polymorphisms operates early in the disease process and requires the presence of *H. pylori* infection. When *H. pylori* attaches to the gastric mucosa, a vigorous inflammatory response with a high IL-1β/TNF-α component may appear to be beneficial in driving the infection out, but concomitant inhibition of acid secretion may allow the infection to extend its colonization and damaging inflammation to the corpus mucosa, an area that is usually well protected by secretion of acid. Future goals of gastric cancer genetic studies include further investigation of key tumor suppressor pathways (e.g., p16/cyclin D1/Rb), development of genetic alterations in gastric cancer, and examination of gene and protein expression patterns in dysplastic and cancerous tissue [38, 39, 40].

Researchers are beginning to identify genetic factors that contribute to the development of gastric cancer in some individuals. Specifically, the E-cadherin gene (CDH1) has been associated with a high risk of gastric cancer. Hereditary diffuse gastric cancer is a rare and deadly form of gastric cancer that can result from CDH1 mutations. Parents who carry this genetic mutation have a 50% chance of passing it along to their offspring. Three out of four people who inherit this genetic mutation will eventually develop gastric cancer [38, 39, 40].

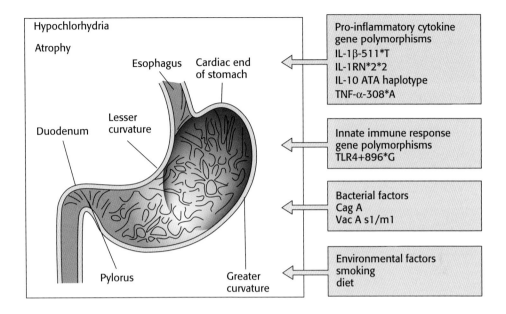

Figure 8.1. Host factors contributing to *H. pylori*-related gastric cancer. From McKinlay AW, El-Omar E. Adenocarcinoma (gastric cancer and miscellaneous malignancy). In Weinstein WM, Hawkey CJ and Bosch J eds., *Clinical Gastroenterology and Hepatology*. New York: Elsevier Mosby, 2005; pp. 233–42, Figure 37.1, p. 235.

High-magnification endoscopy

Early gastric carcinoma is primarily detected and diagnosed by endoscopic examination with or without biopsy. In general, the diagnosis of early gastric carcinoma is easily accomplished by endoscopic observation and pathologic evaluation of the endoscopic biopsy. Endoscopic detection of gastric carcinoma depends on recognition of visible mucosal changes. High-magnification endoscopy (Figure 8.2a) offers the potential to visualize these changes earlier by virtue of its ability to depict the surface mucosal pattern (pit pattern) and capillary structures of the gastric epithelium and lamina propria [1, 41].

Based on analysis of the mucosal pit pattern obtained by magnification, histologic changes of carcinoma, dysplasia, and adenoma can be suspected. However, it is not always easy to diagnose the histologic changes from the magnification pictures. In addition, the entire gastric mucosa wall is difficult to scan with magnified images. Thus the role of high-magnification endoscopy is to magnify a target area in which conventional endoscopy detects an abnormality. This is assisted by dye

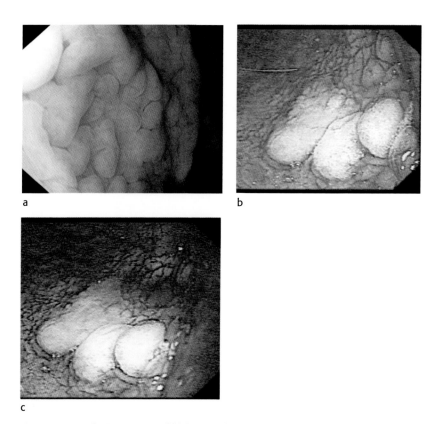

a   b

c

Figure 8.2a–c. The importance of high-magnification upper gastrointestinal endoscopy and chromoendoscopy in detecting early gastric cancers. (a) High-magnification endoscopy can depict the surface mucosal pattern (pit pattern) and capillary structures of the gastric wall. Tumors are better appreciated after spraying them with indigo carmine dye (b) or Lugol's solution (c).

spraying (see Chapter 2) with indigo carmine dye (Figure 8.2b) and Lugol's solution (Figure 8.2c) for gastric carcinoma [1, 41].

Optical coherence tomography

Optical coherence tomography (OCT) is an optical imaging modality (Figure 8.3) that performs high-resolution, cross-sectional, subsurface tomographic imaging of the microstructure of tissues. The physical principle of OCT is similar to that of B-mode ultrasound imaging, except that it uses infrared light waves rather than acoustic waves. The in vivo resolution is 10–25 times better (about 10 µm) than with high-frequency ultrasound imaging, but the depth of penetration is limited to

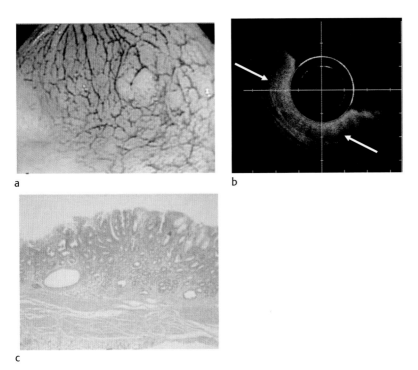

a b

c

Figure 8.3a–c. Optical coherence tomography with endoscopic–pathologic correlation in a patient with Type IIA early gastric cancer. (a) Endoscopic view with indigo carmine dye spraying shows a focal mucosal mass. (b) This lesion is depicted as mass (arrows) which disrupts the normal stratification of the gastric wall on optical coherence tomography. (c) Mucosectomy material reveals well-differentiated adenocarcinoma limited to the mucosa.

1–3 mm, depending upon tissue structure, depth of focus of the probe used, and pressure applied to the tissue surface [41, 42, 43, 44, 45, 46, 47, 48].

Since the late 1990s, OCT technology has evolved from an experimental laboratory tool to a new diagnostic imaging modality with a wide spectrum of clinical applications, including the GI tract and pancreatic-biliary ductal system. OCT imaging from the GI tract can be done in humans by using narrow-diameter, catheter-based probes that can be inserted through the accessory channel of either a conventional front-view endoscope, for investigating the epithelial structure of the GI tract, or a side-view endoscope inside a standard endoscopic retrograde cholangiopancreatography (ERCP) catheter, for investigating the pancreaticobiliary ductal system.

The esophagus and the gastroesophageal junction are the organs most widely investigated to date. More recently, the stomach, duodenum, colon, and pancreaticobiliary ductal system have been extensively investigated. OCT imaging of the gut wall shows a multiple-layer architecture that permits an accurate evaluation of the mucosa, lamina propria, muscularis mucosa, and part of the submucosa. The technique may be used to identify pre-neoplastic conditions of the GI tract, such as Barrett epithelium and dysplasia, and evaluate the depth of penetration of early-stage neoplastic lesions.

In a study [45] of 26 cases of GI tract diseases, including 2 cases of early esophageal carcinoma, 14 of early gastric carcinoma, and 1 of early duodenal carcinoma, all lesions were demonstrated by EOCT with high resolution but poor penetration. The depth of imaging penetration was 1.5–2.0 mm, but the mucosal glandular structure could not be demonstrated. The lamina propria, muscularis mucosa, and part of the submucosa were all well depicted. The gastric wall was observed as a layered structure. The surface layer showed a glandular structure. Deep to the epithelium are three layers which represent the lamina propria (high reflectivity), muscularis mucosa (low reflectivity), and interface layer of submucosal tissue (high reflectivity). Though the resolution was much higher than that of the 30-MHz US scanner, the penetration achieved by EOCT was too poor to use this method to assess the depth of tumor invasion. However, by using this sophisticated instrument, the histologic nature of tissues was demonstrated. EOCT, if perfected, might be used as a method for optical biopsy in the future along with the endoscopic examination.

Sentinel node navigation surgery

Stage I gastric cancer accounts for approximately 61% of all surgically resected cases in Japan. Because lymph node metastases occur in only 10%–16% of patients with early gastric cancer, reduction or omission of a D2 lymphadenectomy would be beneficial if it were possible to predict the extent of lymph node metastases in each patient [49, 50, 51, 52, 53, 54, 55].

Sentinel node navigation surgery (SNNS) is now widely available as reduction surgery for cancers of the breast, colon and rectum, prostate, lung and female genital tract. A sentinel node (SN) is defined as the lymph node that is first to receive the flow of lymphatic fluid from the area containing the primary tumor of an organ. According to the SN hypothesis, lymph node dissection can be omitted when no metastases are detected in SNs. Sentinel lymphatic stations (SLS) represent all the lymphatic stations to which SNs belong (Figure 8.4).

Sentinel node identification is performed with radioactive tin colloid and/or indocyanine green (ICG). Some 2 ml of technetium-99m tin colloid (74 MBq/ml) is injected into the submucosa of the stomach at four sites around the tumor 21 h

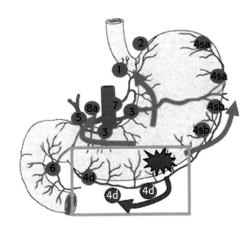

Tumor

Sentinel node

Non-sentinel node

Sentinel lymphatic station

Figure 8.4. Concepts of sentinel node (SN) and sentinel lymphatic station (SLS) in patients with gastric cancer. Numbers represent lymphatic stations, which are defined in the Japanese Classification of Gastric Carcinoma (see Chapter 7). Perigastric lymphatic stations are classified as numbers 1–6. If 2 SNs are identified in lymphatic station number 4d (blue), and number 4d contains not only these SNs but also another non-SN (red), these 3 nodes are regarded as belonging to the SLS. The precise sentinel node depends on the location of the gastric cancer within the stomach. Lymph node stations: 1 = right paracardiac; 2 = left paracardiac; 3 = lesser curvature; 4sa = short gastric; 4sb = left gastroepiploic; 4d = right gastroepiploic; 5 = suprapyloric; 6 = infrapyloric; 7 = left gastric artery; 8a = left common hepatic artery.

before surgery. Just after laparotomy, 4 ml of 1.25% indocyanine green is delivered endoscopically into the same areas as the radiocolloid injection. A hand-held gamma-detector probe is used to identify hot nodes and guide the surgery interoperatively. An SN is any hot node whose ex vivo radioactivity is at least 10 times higher than the background count and/or any node in which green dye uptake is visualized.

In one series [51], the SN concept held true at the occult metastasis level in 96% of patients with gastric cancer, and the accuracy of SNNS was elevated to 100% by using the SLS. If there are no metastases in SNs in SLSs, no further dissection is necessary. They also found that the possibility of metastasis beyond the SLS is low if there are no lymph nodes > 2 mm in diameter in the SLS.

Indocyanine green (ICG) fluorescent imaging (Figures 8.5 and 8.6) is a very promising technique which allows intraoperative lymph node visualization when the ICG is injected the day before surgery.

Perfusion imaging

Pathologic TNM staging, histologic grading, serosal involvement, and lymphatic and solid organ metastasis have all been identified as important predictors of

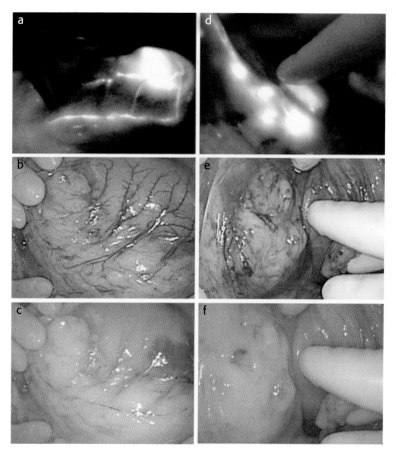

Figure 8.5a–f. The indocyanine green (ICG) fluorescent imaging system clearly visualizes lymphatic vessels from the primary gastric tumor leading towards the lymph nodes. Fine lymph vessels colored faint green (b) are easier to recognize by ICG fluorescent imaging (a) or infrared (IR) imaging (c). Lymph nodes barely perceptible by the green color only (e) are also easier to identify through fat by fluorescent (d) or IR imaging (f). In this patient, the fluorescent imaging system clearly visualizes the four nodes at station number 6 (d), although the IR imaging videoscope (f) does not. From Miyashiro I, Miyoshi N, Hiratsuka M *et al.* Detection of sentinel node in gastric surgery by indocyanine green fluorescence imaging: comparison with infrared imaging. *Ann Surg Oncol* 15: 1640–3, 2008, Figure 1a–f.

prognosis in patients with gastric cancer. One additional factor, tumor microvessel density (MVD), is a very important prognostic tool as well. This factor measures angiogenesis, which is a highly complex process in which new blood vessels develop, generating a new blood supply that is essential for the growth of solid tumors. These new blood vessels enable rapid tumor growth and increase the potential for tumor metastases. MVD, which can be assessed on biopsy and surgical specimen material, may demonstrate intraluminal cancer cells in up to 15% of tumor blood vessels. It is

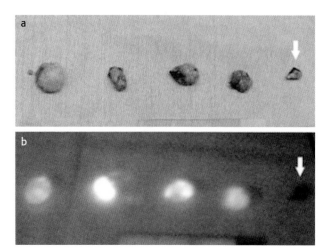

Figure 8.6a,b. Fluorescent imaging confirming that excised lymph nodes stain with ICG; same patient as Figure 8.5. Lymph nodes viewed with normal light (a) and fluorescence (b). The arrows indicate a negative control lymph node from station number 4sb, which was recognized at the time of surgery as a non-sentinel lymph node by the green color, IR imaging videoscope, and the ICG fluorescent imaging system. From Miyashiro I, Miyoshi N, Hiratsuka M *et al.* **Detection of sentinel node in gastric surgery by indocyanine green fluorescence imaging: comparison with infrared imaging.** *Ann Surg Oncol* **15: 1640–3, 2008, page 1643, Figure 2a,b.**

proposed that these small, leaky vessels permit tumor cells to reach the circulatory system, thus increasing the probability of hematogenous metastases [52, 53, 54, 55, 56, 57, 58].

Recent advances in MDCT have made perfusion imaging, a noninvasive means of estimating tumor angiogenesis and permeability, a reality. This method has been successful in assessing tumor vascular physiology and predicting vascular invasion and metastases in brain, lung, liver, neck, and breast neoplasms and also has been used for tumor risk stratification and monitoring tumor response to the therapy [52, 53, 54, 55, 56, 57, 58].

At the present time, perfusion CT is calculated by the deconvolutional approach, which is based on the theory that immediate tumor enhancement is secondary to the presence of contrast medium within the intravascular space and its first-pass into the extravascular space. Tumor enhancement results from the presence of contrast medium in both the intravascular and extravascular spaces. The deconvolutional model has the ability to tolerate greater image noise and as a result is well suited to abdominal scans, particularly gastric cancers, which generally have low levels of perfusion [55, 56, 57, 58].

Perfusion imaging (Figure 8.7) can assess tumor blood flow (BF), blood volume (BV), mean transit time of contrast medium (MTT), and permeability

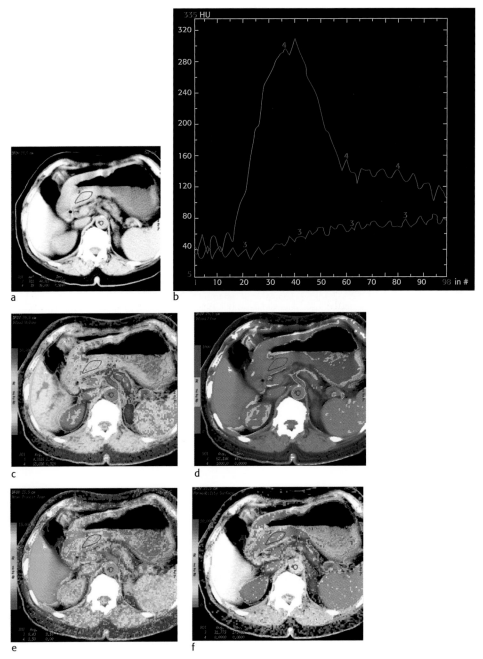

Figure 8.7a–f. MDCT perfusion imaging of a poorly differentiated Bormann Type III gastric cancer. (a) Axial image prior to contrast administration reveals an ulcerated antral mass. (b) Corresponding time density curves show arterial and tumor attenuation change with time. (c) Image calculating blood volume with mean value of 4.33/100 g per min. (d) Image calculating blood flow with a mean value of 62.20 ml/100 g per min. (e) Image calculating mean transit time of 8.49 s, which is rather low. (f) Permeability surface was high with a mean of 31.77 ml/100 g per min.

surface (PS). Zhang *et al.* [59] determined that PS was the only significant prognostic factor in predicting patients with lymph node metastases. PS represents the transmission rate of the contrast medium from capillary endothelium to the interstitial space, and reflects the integrity of endothelial cells and permeability of vessels. As a rule, tumor capillaries have wider inter-endothelial junctions, a large number of fenestrations and transendothelial canals, and a discontinuous or absent basement membrane. These are more easily penetrated by large particles, including tumor cells, when compared to normal blood vessels. This entire process often occurs with an inflammatory reaction that accelerates permeability changes.

Conclusion

Cancer of the stomach remains a common and deadly malignancy. It is interesting to note that although Napoleon's risk factors and family history are better understood now, it is unlikely that his gastric cancer would have been found earlier despite tremendous strides in radiologic and endoscopic imaging. Accordingly, it is doubtful whether his chances of survival would have been greater than 10% in view of the advanced nature of his tumor even with state-of-the-art surgery, chemotherapy, and radiation therapy. This emphasizes the importance of prevention and early detection, and these can only be achieved through advances in understanding of the pathogenesis of this tumor [1].

REFERENCES

1. McKinlay and El-Omar EM. Adenocarcinoma (gastric cancer and miscellaneous malignancy). In Weinstein WM, Hawkey CJ, and Bosch J eds., *Clinical Gastroenterology and Hepatology*. Philadelphia, PA: Elsevier-Mosby, 2005; pp. 233–42.
2. Waxman I and Parmar KS. Clinical aspects and management of gastric carcinoma: diagnostic and staging procedures. In Abbruzzese JL, Evans DB, Willett CG, and Fenoglio-Preiser C eds., *Gastrointestinal Oncology*. New York: Oxford University Press, 2004; pp. 294–301.
3. Stomach. In *World Cancer Research Fund, American Institute for Cancer Research: Food, Nutrition and the Prevention of Cancer: A Global Perspective*. Washington DC: The Institute, 1997; pp. 148–75.
4. Buiatti E, Palli D, Decarli A *et al.* A case-control study of gastric cancer and diet in Italy: II. Association with nutrients. *Int J Cancer* 1990; **45**(5): 896–901.
5. Blot WJ, Li JY, Taylor PR *et al.* Nutrition intervention trials in Linxian, China: supplementation with specific vitamin/mineral combinations, cancer incidence, and disease-specific mortality in the general population. *J Natl Cancer Inst* 1993; **85**(18): 1483–92.

6. Plummer M, Vivas J, Lopez G *et al*. Chemoprevention of precancerous gastric lesions with antioxidant vitamin supplementation: a randomized trial in a high-risk population. *J Natl Cancer Inst* 2007; **99**(2): 137–46.

7. Taylor PR. Prevention of gastric cancer: a miss. *J Natl Cancer Inst* 2007; **99**(2): 101–3.

8. Malila N, Taylor PR, Virtanen MJ *et al*. Effects of alpha-tocopherol and beta-carotene supplementation on gastric cancer incidence in male smokers (ATBC Study, Finland). *Cancer Causes Control* 2002; **13**(7): 617–23.

9. Correa P, Fontham ET, Bravo JC *et al*. Chemoprevention of gastric dysplasia: randomized trial of antioxidant supplements and anti-*Helicobacter pylori* therapy. *J Natl Cancer Inst* 2000; **92**(23): 1881–8.

10. Wong BC, Lam SK, Wong WM *et al*. *Helicobacter pylori* eradication to prevent gastric cancer in a high-risk region of China: a randomized controlled trial. *J Am Med Assoc* 2004; **291**(2): 187–94.

11. Nomura A, Stemmermann GN, Chyou PH *et al*. *Helicobacter pylori* infection and gastric carcinoma among Japanese Americans in Hawaii. *N Engl J Med* 1991; **325**(16): 1132–6.

12. Parsonnet J, Friedman GD, Vandersteen DP *et al*. *Helicobacter pylori* infection and the risk of gastric carcinoma. *N Engl J Med* 1991; **325**(16): 1127–31.

13. Forman D, Newell DG, Fullerton F *et al*. Association between infection with *Helicobacter pylori* and risk of gastric cancer: evidence from a prospective investigation. *Br Med J* 1991; **302**(6788): 1302–5.

14. Parsonnet J, Harris RA, Hack HM *et al*. Modelling cost-effectiveness of *Helicobacter pylori* screening to prevent gastric cancer: a mandate for clinical trials. *Lancet* 1996; **348**(9021): 150–4.

15. Miehlke S, Kirsch C, Dragosics B *et al*. *Helicobacter pylori* and gastric cancer: current status of the Austrian Czech German gastric cancer prevention trial (PRISMA Study). *World J Gastroenterol* 2001; **7**(2): 243–7.

16. Cheung TK, Xia HH, and Wong BC. *Helicobacter pylori* eradication for gastric cancer prevention. *J Gastroenterol* 2007; **42** (Suppl 17): 10–15.

17. de Vries AC, Haringsma J, and Kuipers EJ. The detection, surveillance and treatment of premalignant gastric lesions related to *Helicobacter pylori* infection. *Helicobacter* 2007; **12**(1): 1–15.

18. Jessup JM. Therapeutic principles of gastrointestinal neoplasia: emerging therapies: vaccines. In Abbruzzese JL, Evans DB, Willett CG, and Fenoglio-Preiser C eds., *Gastrointestinal Oncology*. New York: Oxford University Press, 2004; pp. 102–11.

19. Lee Y-C, Lin J-T, Chen T, and Wu M-S. Is eradication of *Helicobacter pylori* the feasible way to prevent gastric cancer? New evidence and progress, but still a long way to go. *J Formos Med Assoc J* 2008; **107**: 591–9.

20. Tahara E. Molecular biology of gastric cancer. In Abbruzzese JL, Evans DB, Willett CG, and Fenoglio-Preiser C eds., *Gastrointestinal Oncology*. New York: Oxford University Press, 2004; pp. 268–80.

21. Hisamuchi S, Fukao P, Sugawara N *et al*. Evaluation of mass screening programme for stomach cancer in Japan. In Miller AB, Chamberlain J, Day NE *et al*. eds., *Cancer Screening*. Cambridge University Press, 1991; pp. 357–72.

22. Hamashima C, Shibuya D, Yamazaki H *et al*. The Japanese guidelines for gastric cancer screening. *Jpn J Clin Oncol* 2008; **38**: 259–67.
23. Kampschöer GH, Fujii A, and Masuda Y. Gastric cancer detected by mass survey. Comparison between mass survey and outpatient detection. *Scand J Gastroenterol* 1989; **24**(7): 813–17.
24. Oshima A, Hirata N, Ubukata T *et al*. Evaluation of a mass screening program for stomach cancer with a case-control study design. *Int J Cancer* 1986; **38**(6): 829–33.
25. Hirayama T, Hisamichi S, Fujimoto I *et al*. Screening for gastric cancer. In Miller AB ed., *Screening for Cancer*. New York: Academic Press, 1985; pp. 367–76.
26. Tytgat GN, Mathus-Vliegen EM, and Offerhaus J. Value of endoscopy in the surveillance of high-risk groups for gastrointestinal cancer. In Sherlock P, Morson BC, Barbara L *et al*. eds., *Precancerous Lesions of the Gastrointestinal Tract*. New York: Raven Press, 1983; pp. 305–18.
27. Inaba S, Hirayama H, Nagata C *et al*. Evaluation of a screening program on reduction of gastric cancer mortality in Japan: preliminary results from a cohort study. *Prev Med* 1999; **29**(2): 102–6.
28. Mizoue T, Yoshimura T, Tokui N *et al*. Prospective study of screening for stomach cancer in Japan. *Int J Cancer* 2003; **106**(1): 103–7.
29. Riecken B, Pfeiffer R, Ma JL *et al*. No impact of repeated endoscopic screens on gastric cancer mortality in a prospectively followed Chinese population at high risk. *Prev Med* 2002; **34**(1): 22–8.
30. Pisani P, Oliver WE, Parkin DM *et al*. Case-control study of gastric cancer screening in Venezuela. *Br J Cancer* 1994; **69**(6): 1102–5.
31. Kitahara F, Kobayashi K, Sato T *et al*. Accuracy of screening for gastric cancer using serum pepsinogen concentrations. *Gut* 1999; **44**(5): 693–7.
32. Staël von Holstein C, Eriksson S, Huldt B *et al*. Endoscopic screening during 17 years for gastric stump carcinoma. A prospective clinical trial. *Scand J Gastroenterol* 1991; **26**(10): 1020–6.
33. Ming S and Goldman H. Gastric polyps: a histogenetic classification and its relation to carcinoma. *Cancer* 1965; **18**(6): 721–6.
34. Utsunomiya J, Maki T, Iwama T *et al*. Gastric lesion of familial polyposis coli. *Cancer* 1974; **34**(3): 745–54.
35. Aarnio M, Salovaara R, Aaltonen LA *et al*. Features of gastric cancer in hereditary non-polyposis colorectal cancer syndrome. *Int J Cancer* 1997; **74**(5): 551–5.
36. Kurtz RC and Sherlock P. The diagnosis of gastric cancer. *Semin Oncol* 1985; **12**(1): 11–18.
37. Brenner H, Rothenbacher D, and Arndt V. Epidemiology of stomach cancer. *Methods Mol Biol* 2009; **472**: 467–77.
38. Moss SF and Shirin H. Epidemiology and molecular epidemiology of gastric cancer. In Abbruzzese JL, Evans DB, Willett CG, and Fenoglio-Preiser C eds., *Gastrointestinal Oncology*. New York: Oxford University Press, 2004; pp. 257–67.
39. Fareed KR, Kaye P, Soomro IN *et al*. Biomarkers of response to therapy in oesophago-gastric cancer. *Gut* 2009; **58**(1): 127–43.
40. Carneiro F, Oliveira C, Leite M, and Seruca R. Molecular targets and biological modifiers in gastric cancer. *Semin Diagn Pathol* 2008; **25**(4): 274–87.

41. Yasuda K. Early gastric cancer: diagnosis, treatment techniques and outcomes. *Eur J Gastroenterol Hepatol* 2006; **18**: 839–45.

42. Testoni PA. Optical coherence tomography. *ScientificWorldJournal* 2007; **7**: 87–108.

43. Xiong H, Zeng C, Guo Z *et al.* Potential ability of hematoporphyrin to enhance an optical coherence tomographic image of gastric cancer in vivo in mice. *Phys Med Biol* 2008; **53**(23): 6767–75.

44. Yang VX, Tang SJ, Gordon ML *et al.* Endoscopic Doppler optical coherence tomography in the human GI tract: initial experience. *Gastrointest Endsoc* 2005; **61**(7): 879–90.

45. Shen B and Zuccaro G. Optical coherence tomography in the gastrointestinal tract. *Gastrointest Endosc Clin N Am* 2004; **14**: 555–71.

46. Bouma BE, Tearney GJ, Comptom CC *et al.* High-resolution imaging of the human esophagus and stomach in vivo using optical coherence tomography. *Gastrointest Endosc* 2000; **51**: 467–74.

47. Pfau PR, Sivak MV, Chak A *et al.* Criteria for the diagnosis of dysplasia by endoscopic coherence tomography. *Gastrointest Endosc* 2003; **58**: 196–202.

48. Zuccaro G, Gladkova N, Vargo J *et al.* Optical coherence tomography of the esophagus and proximal stomach in health and disease. *Am J Gastroenterol* 2001; **96**: 2633–9.

49. Tajima Y, Yamazaki K, Masuda Y *et al.* Sentinel node mapping guided by indocyanine green fluorescence imaging in gastric cancer. *Ann Surg* 2009; **249**: 58–62.

50. Kusano M, Tajima Y, Yamazaki K *et al.* Sentinel node mapping guided by indocyanine green fluorescence imaging: a new method for sentinel node navigation surgery in gastrointestinal cancer. *Dig Surg* 2008; **25**: 103–8.

51. Miyashiro I, Miyoshi N, Hiratsuka M *et al.* Detection of sentinel node in gastric cancer surgery by indocyanine green fluorescence imaging: comparison with infrared imaging. *Ann Surg Oncol* 2008; **15**(6): 1640–3.

52. Morita D, Tsuda H, Ichikura T *et al.* Analysis of sentinel node involvement in gastric cancer. *Clin Gastroenterol Hepatol* 2007; **5**: 1046–52.

53. Bergers G and Benjamin LE. Tumorigenesis and the angiogenic switch. *Nat Rev Cancer* 2003; **3**: 401–10.

54. Fox SB. Tumor angiogenesis and prognosis. *Histopathology* 1997; **30**: 294–301.

55. Miles KA and Griffiths MR. Perfusion CT: a worthwhile enhancement. *Br J Radiol* 2003; **76**: 220–31.

56. Kee TY, Purdie TG, and Stewart E. CT imaging of angiogenesis. *Q J Nucl Med* 2003; **47**: 171–87.

57. Sanelli PC, Nicola G, Tsiouris AJ *et al.* Reproducibility of postprocessing of quantitative CT perfusion maps. *AJR Am J Roentgenol* 2007; **188**: 213–18.

58. d'Assignies G, Couvelard A, Bahrami S *et al.* Pancreatic endocrine tumors: tumor blood flow assessed with perfusion CT reflects angiogenesis and correlates with prognostic factors. *Radiology* 2009; **250**: 407–16.

59. Zhang J, Pan Z, Du L *et al.* Advanced gastric cancer and perfusion imaging using multidetector row computed tomography: correlation with prognostic determinants. *Korean J Radiol* 2008; **9**: 119–27.

Index